THE KHARTOUM MEDICAL STUDENTS' ASSOCIATION

FIFTY YEARS OF OUTSTANDING ACHIEVEMENTS:

1954 - 2005

THE KHARTOUM MEDICAL STUDENTS' ASSOCIATION

FIFTY YEARS OF OUTSTANDING ACHIEVEMENTS:
1954 - 2005

DR AHMED MSK HASHIM

YOUCAXTON PUBLICATIONS

OXFORD AND SHREWSBURY

ISBN 978-1-911175-90-2
Published by YouCaxton Publications 2017

YouCaxton Publications
enquiries@youcaxton.co.uk

First of all, I would like to thank God for giving me the inspiration, guidance, strength and patience to complete this work

This work is dedicated to my mother, for her endless love, support and encouragement throughout my life.

To my father and brother for their guidance and support.

Foreword

This is a unique and fascinating book. It documents the evolution of a student body in the medical school of Khartoum over 50 years. The book narrates the events in a very stimulating manner that compels the reader to remain hooked to the pages until one goes through the whole book. It gives the generations of the medical students who were executives of the association and indeed, all of the students who enjoyed those golden years a nostalgia which refreshes their minds and souls of those happy years. This documentation is absolutely required.

The extra-curricular activities of students in various fields so nicely presented assure leading role of the medical school of Khartoum at a time well ahead of later contemporaries.

The book covers in pictures and legends many events both in the premises of the faculty and places far away in the Sudan. The author must have done a great effort gathering these interesting photos.

I enjoyed the reading of this stimulating book and found great pleasure in going back into history of a most joyful period in my life. I am sure most readers will feel the same.

I congratulate my student Ahmed on this remarkable achievement.

Professor Abdelrahman M. Musa (FRCP)
Professor of Medicine

Contents

List of Abbreviations

EDC	Education Development Centre
FAMSA	Federation of African Medical Students' Association
GA	General Assembly
IFMSA	International Federation of Medical Students' Associations
KMSA	Khartoum Medical Students' Association
KUSU	Khartoum University Students' Union
MedSIN-Sudan	Medical Students' International Network - Sudan
MSA	Medical Students' Association
SCOPA	Standing Committee on Population Activities
SCOPH	Standing Committee on Public Health
SCOR	Standing Committee on Refugees
SCORP	Standing Committee on Refugees & Peace
SMM	Sudan Medical Missions
SMS	Students' Medical Society
SMSA	Sudan Medical Students' Association
SweMSIC	Swedish Medical Students' International Committee
SIDA	Swedish International Development Agency
U of K	University of Khartoum
VCP	Village Concept Project
WHO	World Health Organisation
UNICEF	United Nations International Children's Emergency Fund
WNTD	World No Tobacco Day
WPD	World Peace Day

Introduction & Acknowledgement

MEDICAL STUDENTS at the University of Khartoum are well known for their enthusiasm, academic excellence, and hard work, and the Faculty of Medicine there claims to admit the brightest and most ambitious students in Sudan. The competition for entry to the medical school becomes more challenging year by year, as the medical school receives only the top and best-performing students in the rigorous national secondary school certificate exam. Traditionally, these students have been referred to as "The cream of the cream".

Graduates of the Khartoum medical school not only have an outstanding academic profile in medicine but have also excelled in many other fields; its graduates have gone on to become leaders in major organisations, remarkable politicians, famous poets, artists, and even medical lawyers. Since the establishment of the school in 1924, initially as the Kitchener School of Medicine (KSM), Khartoum University medical students have gained exceptional respect from the Sudanese community, being highly regarded individuals in society and treated as academic elites. A typical medical student at this university in its early beginnings would have been an academic scholar as well as a broad-minded and cultured individual, with a genuine interest in the various challenges facing society and ways of addressing them.

The extra-curricular activities of medical students at the University of Khartoum began as early as the 1920s, but it was not until the mid-1950s that an official body (a society and then an association) was created to represent the students and reflect their extra-curricular, as well as academic activities. In the first 50 years after its inception (1954-2004), the Association made numerous outstanding achievements and many social and cultural activities were enjoyed, and community projects initiated by medical students. Locally, medical students were closely connected to the Sudanese community with many politicians, famous artists, poets and musicians visiting the medical school and participating in activities organised by the students within the faculty premises. Nor were their contributions limited to Khartoum University alone, but expanded and extended to both regional and international levels. Medical students from this school took roles and held prestigious positions in many organisations, including African and international medical students' associations.

Despite all these achievements and a history of more than 60 years, the activities of medical students of the University of Khartoum and their experiences in public work outside medicine are not well documented. There have been scattered attempts to write about them, of which the contributions by Prof. Ahmed Elsafi and Dr Ezzan Saeed are the most remarkable, but only as part of general discussions on the history of the school and of medicine in Sudan and were not specifically dedicated to describing the extra-curricular activities of medical students in depth.

This work aims to describe the history of the Khartoum Medical Students' Association (KMSA) in a chronological manner and documents the various activities accomplished by medical students both inside and outside Sudan, with many pictures and photographs included to illustrate these activities. The book concludes by documenting the activities of the 2004-05 term (when the author served as a member of the executive committee) in detail, with a particular focus on the Golden Jubilee celebrations in 2005.

There was no dedicated documentation or archivist team in the early days of the KMSA and this, coupled with many missing documents and lack of continuity due to the suspension of the Association in the 1990s, meant that gathering evidence was not an easy process. The association was subjected to further suspensions recently, and its offices were relocated. This time, the losses were major, as most of the group pictures, dedication plaques, and old documents went missing (according to recent personal communication with the acting steering committee of the association).

The information and events discussed in this book are predominantly based on the efforts of the documentation committee, established in 2004, which the author had the pleasure and joy of heading in preparation for the Association's Golden Jubilee celebrations.

Many of the events described come from personal interviews held with past Association presidents, between 2004 and 2005. Given the lack of authentic documents to back many of the facts mentioned in these interviews, some statements could not be corroborated which has inevitably had an impact on the accuracy of some of the information presented but the author has made every effort to ensure that facts were cross checked and in line with external documents and sources of information to the best of his knowledge.

The other main sources of information used are the past editions of *Al Hakeem* students' journal, the official organ of the student body which contained regular articles on medical faculty news and the KMSA. Other sources have included the medical school website, the International Federation of Medical Students' Associations (IFMSA) newsletters and annual reports, as well as the Federation of African Medical Students' Associations (FAMSA) website. The use of photographs was also emphasised, as these remain good evidence of historical events. Most of these photographs were collected, collated, and identified by the documentation committee (2004-2005) and many were displayed in the Association history museum during the Golden Jubilee celebrations in 2005.

The idea of writing a booklet detailing the history of the medical students' association was proposed at the time of the Golden Jubilee celebrations in 2005. Unfortunately, due to time constraints, the project did not see the light of the day but recently, the Faculty wanted to have a document or chapter written about the history of the students' extra-curricular activities, as part of its international accreditation renewal process. The author was approached by the steering committee of the Association and the idea of writing this book was revived.

This work could have not been achieved without the dedication and enthusiasm of members of the Documentation and Archiving Committee 2004-5: Mohamed Kamaleldin Eltayeb and Mohamed Mustafa. Zuhair Tarig Ismail and Gassan Abdelsalam also made major contributions in the process of collection and labelling of documents. The excellent support given to the committee by Mutaz Elsadig and Ahmed Eltahir (secretary general and president, respectively) at that time was of paramount importance.

Finally, the material in this book relied primarily on the generous contributions and advice received from past presidents and members of the Association and active students; namely Prof. Haddad Karoum, Prof. Abdelrahman Musa, Prof. M.Y. Sukkar, Dr Mirghani A. Abdelaziz, Dr Elsir Hashim, Prof. Ahmed Elsafi, Prof. Abdelrahman Ali, Prof. Mustafa Abdalla Salih, Prof. Mahgoub Abbashar, Mr Tarig Ismail, Dr. Ahmed F. Shadoul, Dr Abdelhadi Abdelgabbar, Dr. Abdelbagi Ahmed, Mr. Nadir Khogali, Dr Haydar Giha, Dr Hamdeen Hammad, Dr Essam Eldin Elamin, Dr Elsadig Askar, Dr Ezzan Saeed Kunna, Dr Elmonzir Bajouri, and Eltahir Abdelrahman

The Beginning of The Khartoum Medical Students' Association (KMSA)

THE KHARTOUM MEDICAL STUDENTS' ASSOCIATION (KMSA), the official representative body of medical students of the University of Khartoum (U of K), was founded during the late years of the British colonial era, in 1954. The first KMSA president, according to the Presidents' Wall of Honour, was Mohamed Ahmed Gabani (**photo 1, also <u>see Appendix</u>**). Some reports suggest that the Society began with the admission of the first batch of medical students to Kitchener School of Medicine (KSM) back in the 1920s. Nonetheless, it appears that the student body was only officially introduced in 1954. The late Professor Haddad Omer Karoum, the second president (personal interview with Prof. Karoum in 2004, **photo 2**), stated that the group did not formally begin their activities until his term, which lasted from 1955-56 and began as a small society known as the Students' Medical Society (SMS) of KSM. Prof. Karoum also mentioned that this organization focused primarily on non-medical issues, namely literature and cultural activities, as well as the students' welfare.

Photo 1 (overleaf): The KMSA's Presidents' Wall of Honour, as it was displayed at the Golden Jubilee Exhibition in 2005. The wall shows (in Arabic) that the first official president was Mohamed Ahmed Gabani (1954-55) followed by Haddad O. Karoum (1955-56).

Note: An error was made here in the order of the presidents of the late 1950s/ early 1960s when the names were copied from the original wall of honour in 2005. The correct order is displayed in the Appendix.

بسم الله الرحمن الرحيم

جامعة الخرطوم

رابطة طلاب كلية الطب

اليوبيل الذهبي

١٩٥٤-٢٠٠٤م

أسماء الرؤساء الذين تعاقبوا على رئاسة الرابطة بالكلية.

٥٥	٥٤	محمد أحمد قبانى
٥٦	٥٥	حداد عمر كروم
٥٧	٥٦	حسن محمد إبراهيم
٥٨	٥٧	محمد عبد العزيز أبو سمرة
٥٩	٥٨	موسى عبد الله حامد
٦٠	٥٩	عبد الرحمن محمد موسى
٦١	٦٠	صلاح طه صالح
٦٢	٦١	
٦٣	٦٢	حسن عثمان عمر
٦٤	٦٣	محمد زين محمد
٦٥	٦٤	عثمان محمد أحمد طه
٦٦	٦٥	على الحاج محمد
٦٧	٦٦	ميرغني أحمد عبد العزيز
٦٨	٦٧	عبد السلام جرجس
٦٩	٦٨	حسن فضل الله
٧٠	٦٩	أحمد إبراهيم مختار
٧١	٧٠	أحمد الصادق
٧٢	٧١	عمر إبراهيم عبود
٧٣	٧٢	محمد المهدى بشير
٧٤	٧٣	عبد الرحمن عبيد
٧٥	٧٤	عبد الماجد محمد مساعد
٧٦	٧٥	بكرى عثمان سعيد

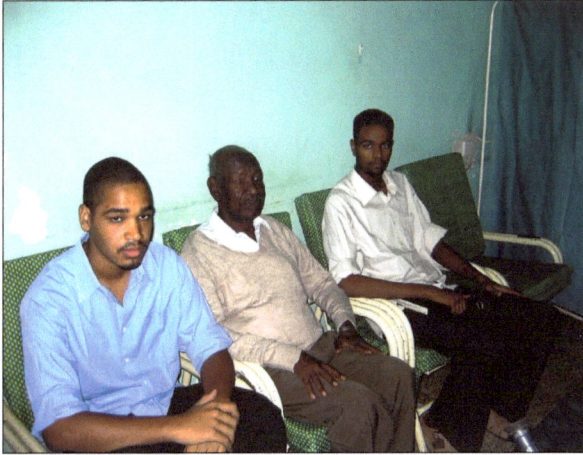

Photo 2: 2004 interview with Prof. Haddad Karoum, Association President 1955-56 (middle). Interview conducted by members of the Documentation and Archiving Committee, Mohamed Kamal (left) and Mohamed Mustafa (right).

It appears that in the early days of the Association, its president was appointed by the faculty dean, with no direct input from the students. When asked about the criteria used to select the president, Prof. Karoum stated that he was appointed because of his good command of English, but as there are no documents from that early period, this cannot be corroborated. Prof. Karoum noted that the president's role at that time was relatively narrow; simply serving as a representative for the student body at major faculty events. Society members' activities were also limited and students published literature in wall magazines.

In **photo 3,** the then-student Haddad Omar Karoum, is shown seated to the far left-hand side of the picture. While not specifically organised by the Students' Society, trips to the countryside were common during that period and one of these is documented in **photo 4,** showing Karoum standing on the right-hand side with another student Nasreldin Ahmed, who is currently a well-known Professor of Physiology and founder of the Khartoum College of

Medical Sciences. Nasreldin is seen third from the right, at the back. Among the other famous students in these photos is Ali Fadul.

Later in the 1950s, the Society held regular annual general meetings (usually in January), during which the annual report of activities was discussed and the new Society committee was elected. By the late 1950s, the committee apparently had 11 members, including seven elected students and four professors (faculty staff members) with the faculty dean acting as Treasurer. It was mainly professor H. V. Morgan, a professor of Internal Medicine and one of the last British deans of the faculty (1955-58), who supervised the Students' Society in those days and acted as its Treasurer. It is not clear what the exact role of each student member was but the major positions given to them were President, Secretary and Editor. The student members of the SMS at that time were elected only from the clinical years, as pre-clinical students stayed within the premises of the main University campus away from the medical school buildings.

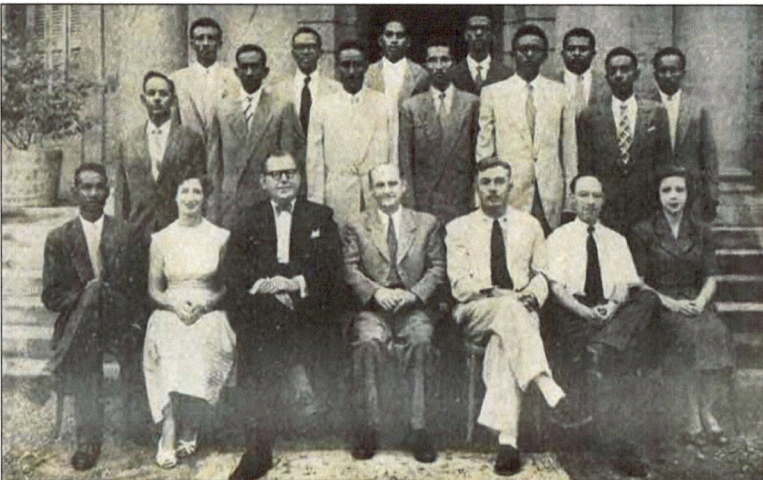

Photo 3: Medical graduates in 1956. Haddad Karoum is seated first from the left. Prof. Morgan is seated in the middle. Nasreldin Ahmed Mohmoud and Ali Fadul are standing in the second row, second and third from the right (respectively) (Source: Faculty of Medicine, U of K website)

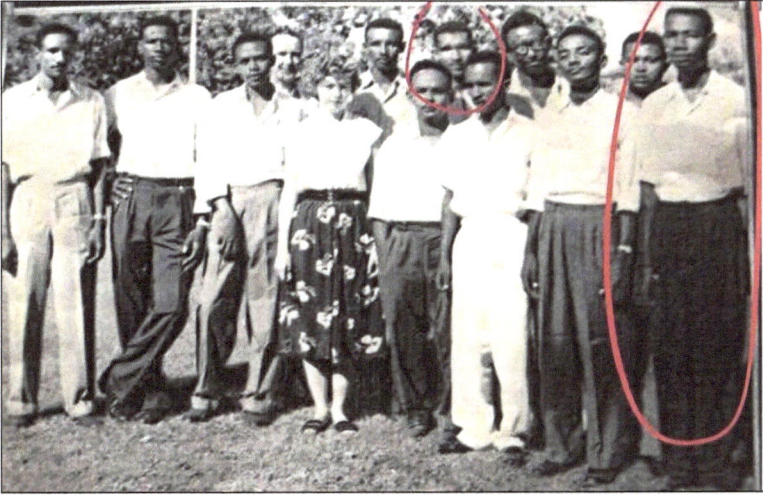

Photo 4: Medical students' field trip, 1955-56. Haddad Karoum, Student Medical Society President, is standing first from the right.

In 1955, a dedicated medical students' magazine was proposed in order to create a platform for showcasing new developments in academic research, as well as student affairs. The first editions were published as wall magazines, but in 1957 the Students' Association decided to take the project further and a print version of the magazine was published.

This magazine was named *Al Hakeem* (also *El Hakeim*), meaning, "doctor or wise person" in traditional Sudanese and the first edition was published in September 1957, under the leadership of Kamal Zaki Mustafa (**photo 5**), who became its first Chief Editor. Professor Morgan remained the main advisory member of the editorial board for *Al Hakeem* for many years and a segment of the *Al Hakeem* archive can be seen in **photo 6**, taken at the Golden Jubilee exhibition. A number of editions were displayed in this exhibition, along with a brief description of the history of the magazine (in Arabic). Originally, *Al Hakeem* was published twice a year and the first few editions were published as *El Hakeim;* this was later changed to *Al Hakeem* in the mid-1960s.

In his editorial of the first edition of *El Hakeim (Al Hakeem)*, Kamal Zaki wrote:

"It honours me to try and introduce to you the first edition of El Hakeim. It took me a lot of time thinking how I am going to launch this newborn and what words I will choose. Just the thought of it gave me the creeps. Finally, I collected the shattered bits of my courage and decided to say: Folks, here it comes!

My dear reader in your hands is a humble attempt of a medical journal. We do not pretend that it is anything near perfection, BUT it is a first trial. We admit that it lacks in many respects, but we strongly believe that with experience and time we will steadily and firmly climb up the ladder. We hope it will not take us too long"

Kamal Zaki was succeeded by Mustafa Khogali in 1958. The magazine then began to appear three times a year, in May, August and December.

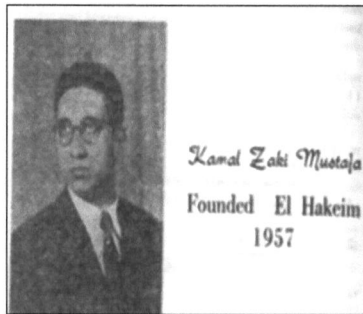

Kamal Zaki Mustafa
Founded El Hakeim
1957

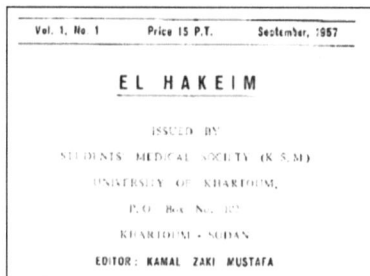

| Vol. 1, No. 1 | Price 15 P.T. | September, 1957 |

EL HAKEIM

ISSUED BY
STUDENTS MEDICAL SOCIETY (K.S.M.)
UNIVERSITY OF KHARTOUM,
P.O. Box No. 127
KHARTOUM - SUDAN
EDITOR: KAMAL ZAKI MUSTAFA

Photo 5: Below: the front page of the first edition of Al Hakeem/El Hakeim journal (Vol. 1. No.1). Above: A portrait of Kamal Zaki Mustafa.

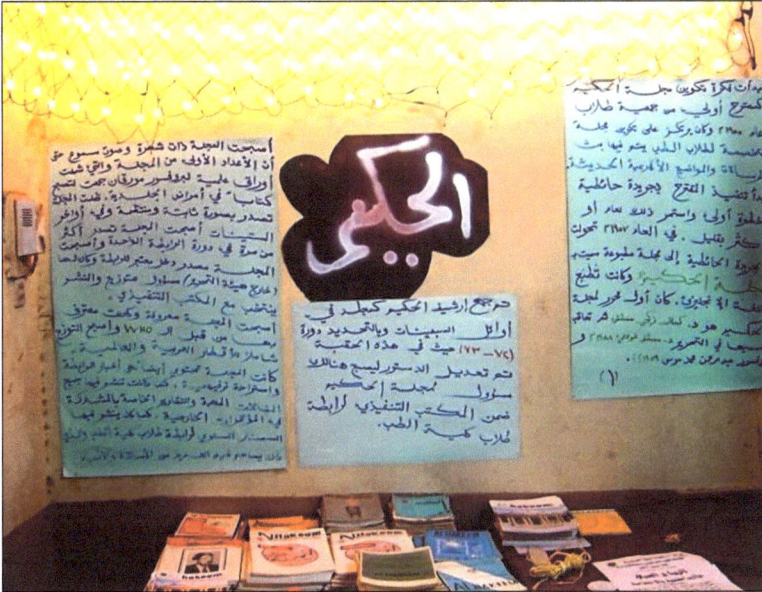

Photo 6: Al Hakeem's archive, as displayed in the Golden Jubilee exhibition, 2005.

In 1959, Abdelrahman Musa became Editor of *Al Hakeem* and put in a lot of effort to maintain the continuity of its publication. The funds allocated to the magazine were limited and Society members approached *Al-Tamaddun* printing house in Khartoum and secured a deal to have *Al Hakeem* printed with deferred payment of printing fees until after the magazine was sold; in exchange for this favour, the students had to physically help in the printing process. Some of those Society committee members of the term 1959-1960 can be seen in **photo 7** which was taken at the old medical students' hostel. Abdelrahman Musa became President of the Society in 1960-61 during which time activities expanded and the Society created its own bank account at Barclay's Bank in Khartoum. He was preceded and succeeded by Musa Abdalla Hamid and Salah Taha Salih respectively.

The Society received generous support from the faculty deans in its early beginnings. According to Prof. Abdelrahman Musa, the routine meetings of the Society members were often held in Prof. Dean Smith's own house. Prof. Smith was the dean of faculty from 1958-60 and the role of the Student Society President also grew in importance during this period, as the president was regularly invited to speak at faculty events. **Photo 8** shows the Students' Society President sitting next to Professor Morgan and, in the bottom image, Musa is seen giving a speech on behalf of the students at the farewell event for Prof. Morgan, who was leaving to work in Ghana. Interestingly, Prof. Morgan decided to return to Sudan only a few weeks after this event.

Al Hakeem was considered to be the first (and leading) student journal of its kind in the country and as such, it inspired other regional student groups to publish their own magazines. Locally, Veterinary students were perhaps the first group to follow in the footsteps of the SMS by publishing their own magazine *El Baittar,* in November 1958, only one year after the inauguration of *Al Hakeem* and the magazine continued to be the official organ of the Veterinary Students' Society, University of Khartoum.

In 1960, Abdelrahman Musa, president of the Society and former editor of *Al Hakeem,* received a letter from the editor of the proposed "Dokita Journal", of the Students' Clinical Society of University College Hospital, Ibadan, Nigeria, in which the editor-to be asked Musa to write a goodwill message, to be published in the Dokita's first issue.

One of the new activities adopted by the Society in the late 1950s were debate sessions, led by the debating group which was formed in 1958 and the first session was held in that year. The idea was supervised and greatly supported by Prof. Lynch, a British professor of Pathology who was passionate to promote the development of social and non-academic skills among students. Lynch later introduced a Prize in Pathology to be awarded to the fourth year medical student who, in addition to academic excellence, demonstrates significant involvement in student social activities.

The Society also published a variety of wall magazines. The most consistent of these was "Cock-tail" displayed in the Kitchener School of Medicine hostel and it published various articles in Arabic. It also occasionally held student photography exhibitions.

Some logistical difficulties faced the Society in organising regular sports activities in the hostels in view of the separation between clinical and pre-clinical years at that time, but it still participated in competitions in major sports such as football, basketball and tennis, held by the University students' union. Medical students often won the tennis tournaments but their football and basketball teams were not that strong.

According to reports in *Al Hakeem,* the Society began to establish networks with regional and international associations in the late 1950s. The general assembly in 1958 accepted recommendations from the executive committee that the SMS should become associate member of the International Federation of Medical Students' Associations (IFMSA). However, this was not implemented until 1966, as will be illustrated in the next chapter. In addition, the SMS proposed the first Pan-African medical students' seminar, perhaps the first ever official attempt to form an African medical student body or platform. A call for this seminar was made by the executive committee of the SMS following its annual meeting in January 1958. Nine medical schools in Africa were invited to participate and were asked to give their input as to the financial and technical aspects. Funding was sought from the International Union of Students and IFMSA. The aims of the seminar as outlined in *Al Hakeem* (Vol.1, No.3) were:

- To promote medical interest among the African medical students.
- Study and exchange of ideas on medical problems of common interest.
- To establish close friendly and professional relations between the different African medical student bodies.
- To seek the common aims and principles of future co-operation.

The preparatory committee of the seminar consisted of four student members, three representatives from the Ministry of Health, the Sudan Medical Association and Khartoum University Students' Union (KUSU). The chairman was the dean of faculty and the Seminar was finally set to take place in July 1959.

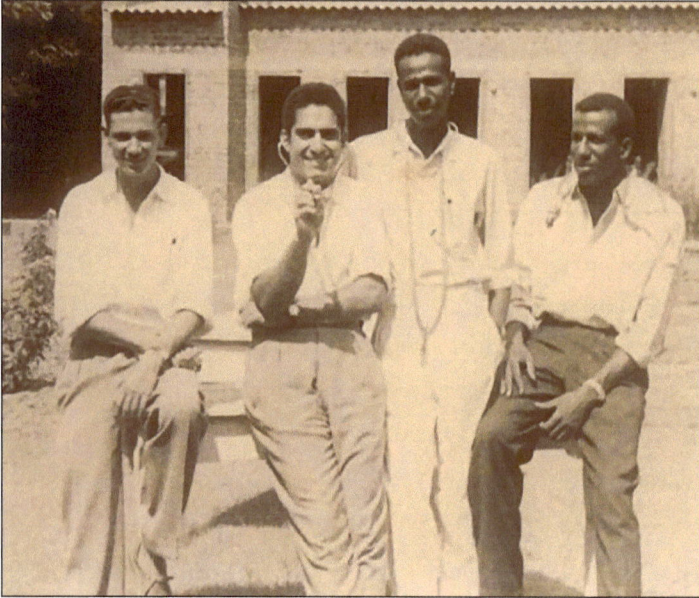

Photo 7: Society committee members, 1959-1960. From right to left: Abdalla Elhag Musa, Abdelrahman Musa, Aasim Zaki Mustafa, M. Yousif Sukkar.

Student community activities were common in the 1950s; students took trips to all parts of the country to undertake community volunteer work and these activities are documented in photographs from that time. Some of the students in these photos later became professors during the so-called Golden Era of Sudanese medicine, including Prof. Mohamed Yousif Sukkar (Professor of Physiology), Prof. Bashir Arbab, Prof. Alsheikh Mahjoub, Mr. Mirghani Sanhoori, and Prof. Abdelrahman Musa.

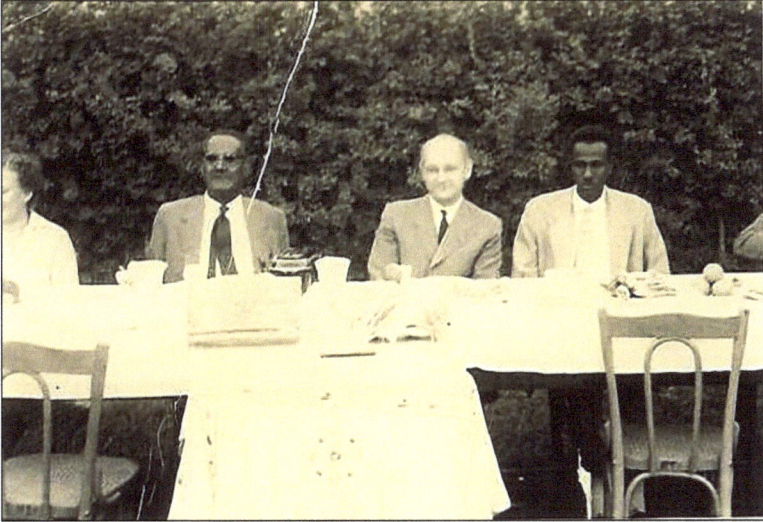

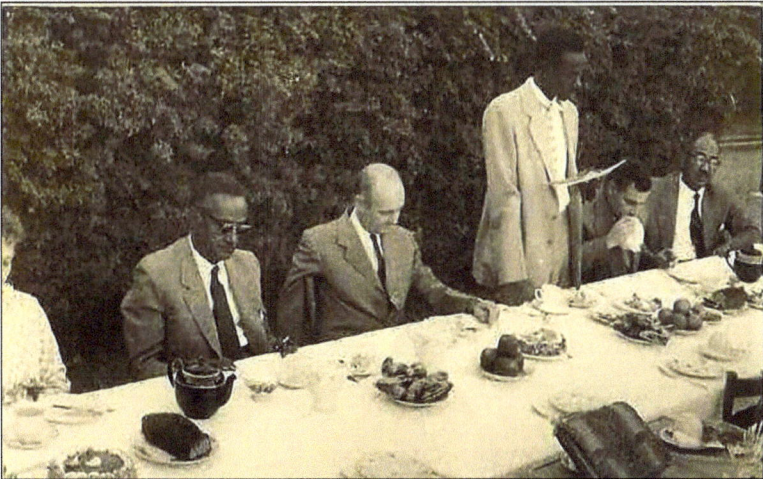

Photo 8: Prof. Morgan's farewell. Top image: Seated first from the right: Abdelrahman Musa, President of the Students' Medical Society (1960-61). Seated in the middle: Prof. Morgan. Seated on the left: Dr. Mohamed Ahmed Ali, Minister of Health. Bottom Image: Abdelrahman Musa is giving a thank-you speech on behalf of the students. To his left sit Prof. Butler (Faculty Dean, 1960-63) and Dr Ahmed Ali Zaki (undersecretary of the Ministry of Health).

The common areas visited in those field tours were Southern Sudan, Kordofan and Nuba Mountains and Darfur, as well as the eastern part of the country, including major cities and towns, such as Port-Sudan and Kassala. The trips were usually supervised by faculty staff from the Department of Preventative (community) Medicine and in addition to their educational value, they seem to have been full of joy, fun and entertainment. Abdelrahman Musa, then Editor of *Al Hakeem,* wrote about various field trips in the year 1959-60. Describing one of the interesting incidents which occurred during their visit to Nuba Mountains in the sixth edition of the journal, Musa wrote:

"Of the most interesting items, I recall our visit to Hagar El Mandal Quarantine, where we were shown cases of small pox among whom was El Kojour himself (El Kojour is the witch doctor of the Nuba). It is sad to note that the disease was brought to the area by one of its natives, who contracted the disease in Port Sudan and travelled hundreds of miles, hiding himself from the health authorities, until he reported in El Kojour's out-patients. The result was that 19 died, among whom was El Kojour's own wife (who was probably Senior Matron). I was explaining to El Kojour that he should not harbour such cases again, but Sukkar, the secretary of Students' Medical Society, passed the word that I was urging El Kojour for an annual subscription to El Hakeim"

In **photo 9**, Professor Anis Mohamed Ali Elshamy, known as the father of community medicine, accompanies students on an outreach trip to explore the role of community intervention and health education in the prevention of Schistosomiasis. The photo shows the students standing behind the barriers which they helped locals to use, in order to prevent the spread of Bilharziasis. A student visit to the Midwifery Hospital in Wed-Medani is documented in **photo 10**, while other medical trips in South Sudan (currently the Republic of South Sudan) are documented in **photo 11** and **12**.

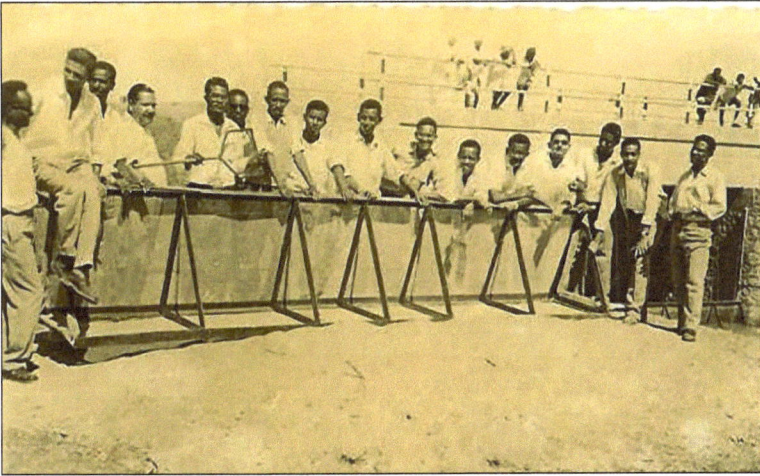

Photo 9: Medical students in Wed-Medani with Anis Elshamy (Professor of Preventative Medicine), 1959. Students are standing behind the barriers they helped locals to use in order to prevent Bilharziasis.

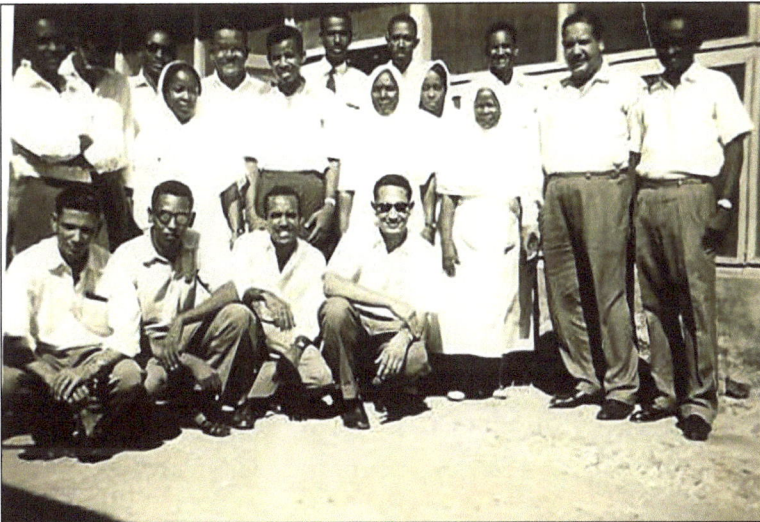

Photo 10: A photo of the same group at the Midwifery Hospital in Wed-Medani. In this photo, Prof. Anis Elshamy is standing second from the right. Students Mohamed Yousif Sukkar (sitting first from the left), Abdelrahman Musa (back row third from the right), Bashir Arbab, and Mirghani Sanhouri can be seen.

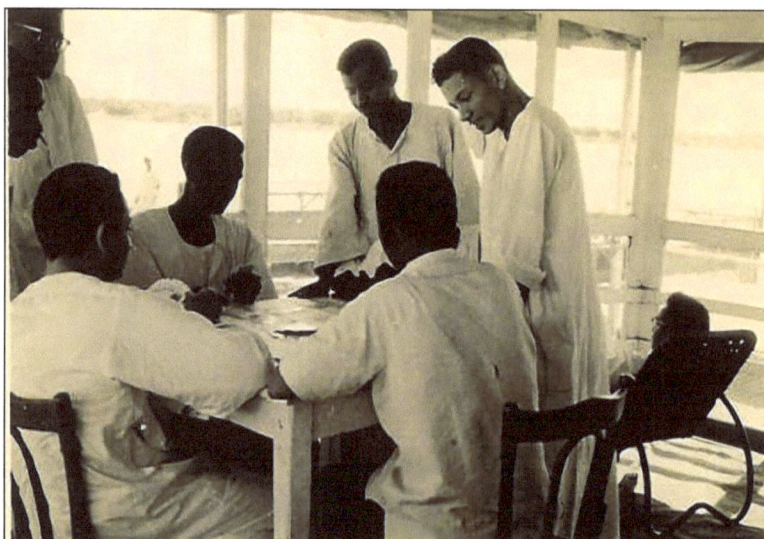

Photo 11: Medical students of the University of Khartoum (U of K) on a boat trip to South Sudan, 1958. M. Y. Sukkar stands first from the right. Other students who appear in this photo are Bashir Arbab and Abdelrahman Musa.

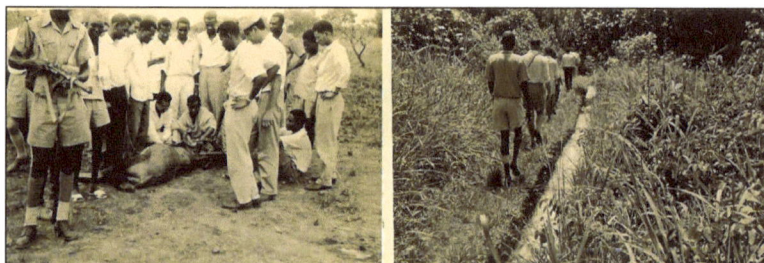

Photo 12: The medical students' field trip to South Sudan, 1958.

The 1960s

The Association Joins International and Regional Student Organisations

In THE 1960s, the Society was restructured to include specific executive roles; Hassan Osman Omer, Mohamed Zain, Osman Mohamed Ahmed Taha, and Ali Elhag Mohammed adopted the role of Society President in succession from 1962-66. At that stage, the executive committee was elected by the students' general assembly, according to specific electoral guidelines, the president being elected from the sixth-year student body, while the Secretary General was elected from the fifth-year students. Professor H. Butler, the last British Dean of the Faculty (1960-63), supervised the Society in the early 1960s.

The elected board consisted of ten members with the following roles:

- President
- Vice-President
- Secretary (General)
- Editor
- Business Manager (Equivalent to financial secretary)
- Advertising Manager
- Distribution (and Sales) Manager
- Three members

and... Four advisory members from the faculty staff, with the faculty dean acting as Treasurer.

Further amendments were made in the late 1960s and the three student members who previously had no official appointment were given the roles of Assistant Secretary, Assistant Editor and Film Show Director.

Al Hakeem continued to be published regularly up to three times a year under supervision by Prof. Morgan and among the prominent editors in the 1960s were the late Salih Yassin, Mustafa Dafaalla, Ahmed Elsafi, Omer Osman Elkhalifa and the late Elfatih Abdalla Hamadein. In recognition of Prof. Morgan's support to the magazine, the Society published a special, dedicated edition of *Al Hakeem* in 1965 (Issue no. 18, January 1965) which included all his scientific articles, particularly those on skin diseases, including 8 articles written by Prof. Morgan on the different aspects of the then newly established discipline of Dermatology. The editor of that term was Elfatih Hamadein.

Following Prof. Morgan's return to the UK in 1968, Dr Makram Girgis kindly accepted to be the Consultant of *Al Hakeem* in Morgan's place. A dedication was written and published in *Al Hakeem* no.23 (Jan 1968) to acknowledge Morgan's contribution to the magazine and his support to the Society activities at large.

In addition, *Al Hakeem* published many social and cultural articles from famous poets and writers. In 1969 the well-known Syrian poet Nizar Gabbani, visited Sudan and was invited by members of the Association to a poetry recital. One of his famous poems at the time *Bread, Hashish and a Moon*, was translated to English by Prof. Eltigani Elmahi and was published in *Al Hakeem* (No. 3 Volume 7) in June 1969, in both Arabic and English versions. In the same edition, the late Mr. Gamal Mohamed Ahmed, a renowned Sudanese scholar and diplomat, wrote a fascinating introduction to the translated version of Nizar's poem.

The years 1966-67 marked a historic time for the Students' Association, with the group widening the scope of its activities in search of international recognition. The Society President then was

Mirghani Ahmed Abdelaziz, and Mohamed Sirelkhatim Hashim (Elsir Hashim) was Secretary General. In personal communications, they both mentioned that the executive committee and the local authorities deliberated extensively before deciding to submit a membership request to the IFMSA. The group's initial hesitations were related to concern over the political situation at the time. The Arab-Israel war had led to government prohibitions preventing Sudanese institutions from joining organisations that recognised Israel as a state.

Nonetheless, an exemption was eventually granted by the Sudanese government and the Students' Society went ahead with its application. However, the exemption process delayed Elsir Hashim's arrival at the IFMSA meeting, which apparently resulted in the inability of the Society's submission to be included formally in the IFMSA GA general agenda. Elsir Hashim finally managed to present the Society's candidature at the IFMSA General Assembly in Athens, in August 1966, where the Society (SMS) was initially granted associate member status and acquired full IFMSA membership the following year. Society members were unable to attend the IFMSA GA in Vienna in 1967 because of acute shortage of money but interestingly, with the help of the Medical Students' Association of the American University of Beirut, the SMS was allowed to attain full membership without attending the GA in person.

Abdelsalam Gerais as business manager and the late Salih Yassin, as editor, were two other notable committee members from that term (1966-67) and their roles are highlighted on the cover page of the 21st issue of the magazine in November 1966 (**photo 13**). Mohamed Sirelkhatim's address to the IFMSA GA was published in the same edition of *Al Hakeem* and a copy of it is displayed below (**photo 14**).

At the end of this term, in its annual meeting in 1967 and following the preliminary acquisition of IFMSA membership, the Society decided on a new, more comprehensive name and the name of the student body was changed from 'Society' to 'Association' (Medical

Students' Association, MSA). Later in the 1970s a further change was made and it became the Sudan Medical Students' Association.

A group photo of the elected board of the Students' Society and faculty advisers from the 1966-67 term is also shown below (**photo 15**). Abdelsalam Gerais became Society President in the following term, from 1967-68.

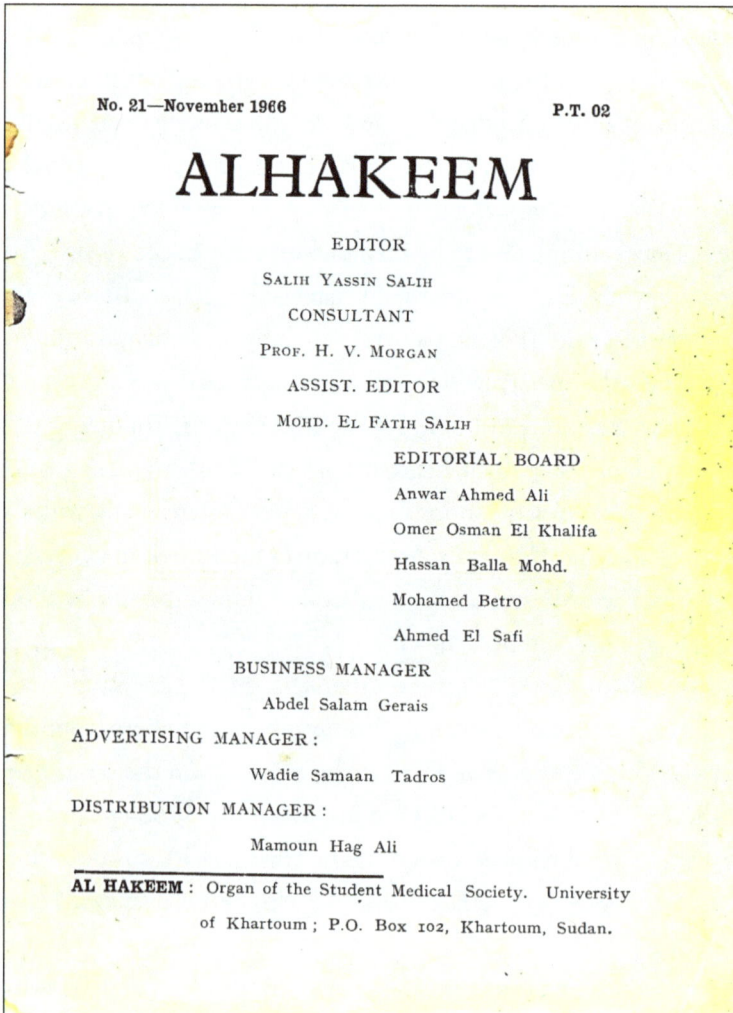

No. 21—November 1966   P.T. 02

ALHAKEEM

EDITOR

SALIH YASSIN SALIH

CONSULTANT

PROF. H. V. MORGAN

ASSIST. EDITOR

MOHD. EL FATIH SALIH

EDITORIAL BOARD

Anwar Ahmed Ali

Omer Osman El Khalifa

Hassan Balla Mohd.

Mohamed Betro

Ahmed El Safi

BUSINESS MANAGER

Abdel Salam Gerais

ADVERTISING MANAGER :

Wadie Samaan Tadros

DISTRIBUTION MANAGER :

Mamoun Hag Ali

AL HAKEEM : Organ of the Student Medical Society. University of Khartoum ; P.O. Box 102, Khartoum, Sudan.

Photo 13: The cover page of Al Hakeem, Nov. 1966 (Editor-in-Chief: Salih Yassin; Advisor: Prof. Morgan; Business Manager: Abdelsalam Gerais).

INTERNATIONAL FEDERATION OF MEDICAL STUDENTS' ASSOCIATIONS

Address of the Delegate of the Sudan, Mr. M. S. Hashim,

to the X Vth General Assembly - Athens 1966

Mr. Chairman, fellow Medical students:

It gives me great pleasure to be here today amongst this distinguished Assembly. I wish to express, on behalf of myself and the Students' Medical Society and the University of Khartoum's Student Union our sincere appreciation for the interest you have shown in our society's participation in this Assembly and in other functions and other activities of the International Federation of the Medical Students' Associations. Now, that we propose for Full-membership in I.F.M.S.A., my Society, looks forwards to effective participation and mutual cooperation.

Allow me, dear friends, to give a brief account of the Society of which I am the Secretary General. The Students' Medical Society of the University of Khartoum was organized in 1954. Initially, the society concerned itself primarily with the welfare of medical students but later, broadened its scope of activities. The Official organ of the Society, "Al-Hakeem" Medical Journal, was established in 1957 and appears regularly three times a year. This Journal is the only one of its kind now published in Sudan.

To further enhance the effectiveness of the Society, annual sominars were started five years ago on the Faculty premisses to discuss and attempt to solve problems of medical importance. Subjects are reviewed, now work is put forward and recommendations are submitted to the authoritis concerned. The participants include the Staff and the Students of our Medical School as well as other faculties, the Staff of Hospitals all over the Country, representatives of the Ministry of Health, private practiotioners and resident W.H.O. Staff. The Main objective of this type of activities is to promote research into medical as well as non-medical fields ; the previous four seminars dealt with :

(1) Infective Hepatitis.

(2) Maternal and Child Welfare.

(3) Development of Medical Education in Sudan.

(4) Schistosomiasis in Sudan.

26

The fifth annual seminar will be held in November, 1966 the subject will be Malnutrition in Sudan.

Mr. Chairman,

Our Society hopes to enlarge its scope even farther we continued to endeavour, to expand and strengthten our relations with similar organizations, beyind the boundaries of our country. It is our sincere hope that our participation in I.F.M.S.A. will enhance the fulfilment of this Objective ; We hope to achieve greater mutual understanding and cooperation. Furthermore, I wish on behalf of the Students' Medical Society of the University of Khartoum, to stress ourinterest in all programmes of I.F.M.S.A. as enumerated in its Publication Introducing I.F.M.S.A., and particularly the one on Professional Exchange. The need of a developing country such as Sudan for further training and professional experience need not be emphasized.

Mr. Chairman, Fellow Medical Students

I wish to convey the greetings and wishes of the President of our Society, Mr. Mirgani Ahmed Abdel Aziz whose unability to be present was the result of our late preparations for this meeting which, unfortunately, was unavoidable ; furthermore the President's active academic programme this final year of his course has made it not possible for him to leave Khartoum.

On behalf of the Students' Medical Society of theUniversity of Khartoum and myself I wish this Assembly all the success in its deliberation.

Thank you

MOHAMED SIREL-KHATIM HASHIM,

Students' Medical Society (U. of K).

I.F.M.S.A. X V General Assembly, August 1966

Athens.

Photo 14: The candidature speech given by Mohamed Sirelkhatim Hashim (Elsir Hashim) at the IFMSA GA in Athens, 1966.

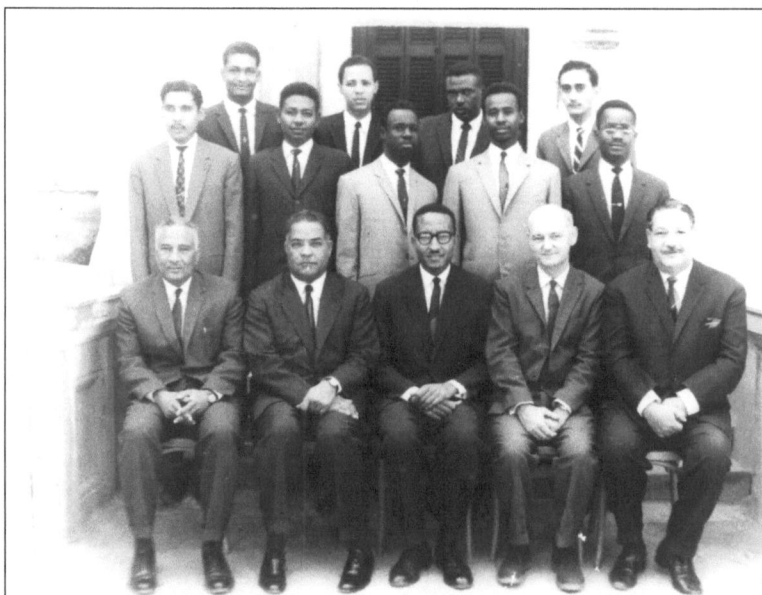

Photo 15: A group picture of the executive board of the Students' Society for the term 1966-67. Seated from left to right: Prof. Daoud Mustafa, Prof. Mansour Ali Haseeb, Mirghani Ahmed Abdelaziz (Society President), Prof. Morgan, Prof. Anis Elshamy. Second row (from left to right): Mohamed Sirelkhatim Hashim (Secretary General), Salih Yassin (Editor of Al Hakeem), Hashim Yagi (Vice-President), Hassan Balla (member), and Abdelsalam Gerais (Business Manager). Back row, from left to right: Hassan Fadlalla (member), Mudather Allam (member), Mamoun Hag Ali (Distribution Manager), Wadie Samaan Tadros (Advertising Manager).

The Society held its first Graduates Day on the 27th of February 1965 and in an interview with Gerais in 2004 (**photo 16**), he said that he and other Society members had organised a second, very successful Graduates Day in 1966, over a period of three days between 27th & 29th of January where graduates, staff and students of the medical school came together and enjoyed a reception tea party, various exhibitions, an evening party and a Gala Night.

The first day was addressed by the Faculty Dean, University Vice-Chancellor, the graduates' representative and the president of the Sudan Medical Association. The next day, faculty staff and graduates went by cars and on foot all the way from the faculty building to the grave of the late Hashim Bey Al-Baghdadi, where they paid tribute to the well-known philanthropist. Al-Baghdadi had donated all his assets to promote the welfare of the medical students and faculty at the U of K (then the Kitchener School of Medicine) and the students and faculty remember him fondly to this day. A lecture theatre and an academic prize are named in his honour.

It is claimed that **photo 17** is from the Graduates Day in 1966, in which Prof. Mansour Ali Haseeb, a professor of microbiology, known for being a pioneer of medical research and the first Sudanese dean of the faculty (1963-69), is laying flowers at the grave of Al-Baghdadi.

The Graduates Day was later replaced by Graduation Day and it remains a student tradition; a celebration organised by the students for the fresh graduates from the Faculty of Medicine.

Prof. Mansour Ali Haseeb, Prof. Daoud Mustafa, and Prof. Morgan remained the main advisers of the Society in the 1960s and were keen promoters and supporters of students' activities. **Photos 15** and **18** show the three of them sitting in the front row, along with the executive members of the society. **Photo 18** is a group picture from one of the Society terms in the mid-1960s (thought to be either the term 1963-64 or 1964-65).

After being accepted into the IFMSA, the Students' Society began participating in numerous international activities. In December 1966, President Mirghani A. Abdel Aziz travelled to Prague to take part in the IFMSA Exchange Officers Meeting (EOM) (**photo 19**). Following the success of this meeting, the Society began to participate officially in the IFMSA professional exchange programme and by the late 1960s, nineteen Sudanese students had joined the exchange programme and travelled to Italy,

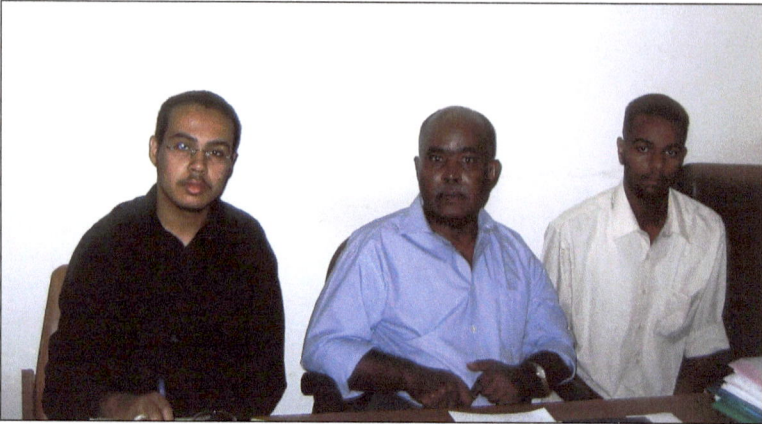

Photo 16: An interview held by the Documentation and Archiving Committee with Prof. Abdelsalam Gerais (Association President 1967-68), Sudan National Centre of Fertility and In Vitro Fertilisation, Khartoum, 2004. From left to right: Ahmed MSK Hashim (Author), Prof. Gerais, Mohamed Mustafa (Documentation Committee member).

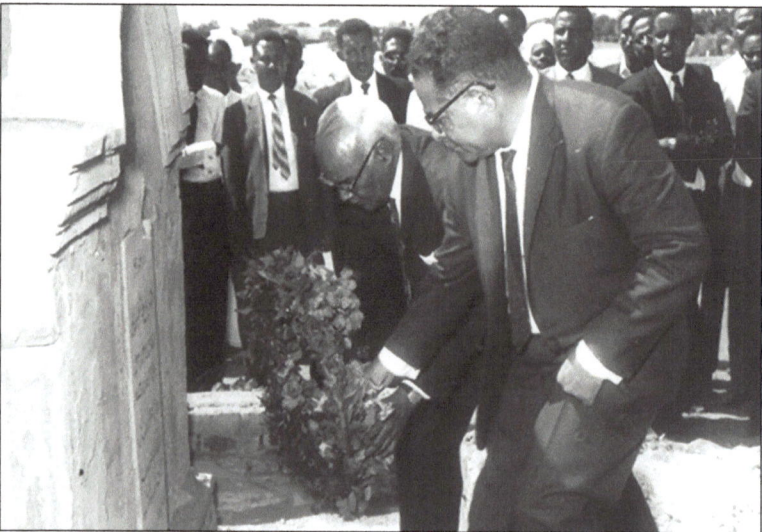

Photo 17: Prof. Haseeb laying flowers at the grave of Hashim Bey Al-Baghdadi (believed to have been taken on the Graduates Day in 1966).

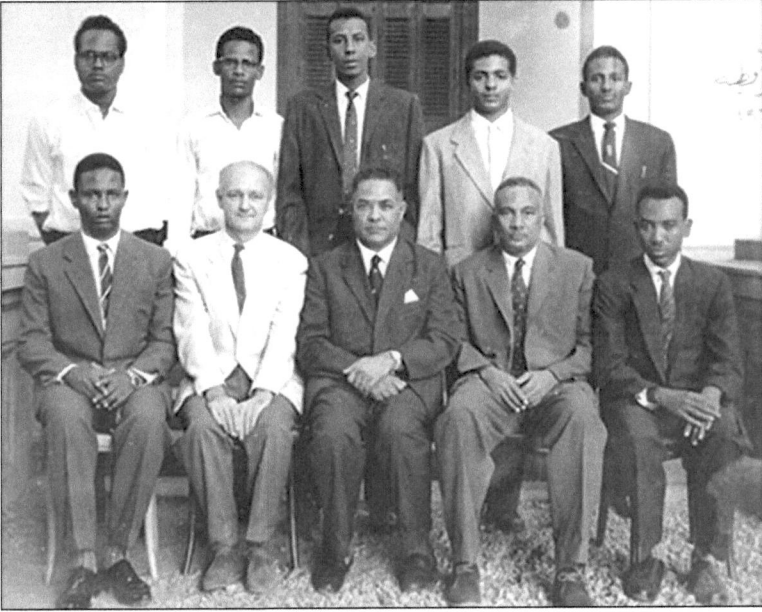

Photo 18: A group picture of the Executive Board of the Students' Medical Society in the mid-1960s. Osman Mohamed Ahmed Taha (Society President, 1964-65) stands in the middle. Mohamed Zain (Society President, 1963-64) is seated first from the right. The late Mustafa Hassan Badeh stands first from the left. Members of the advisory committee, including Prof. Morgan, Prof. Haseeb (Faculty Dean), and Prof. Daoud, are seated in front.

Poland, West Germany, Britain, and Czechoslovakia while seven students were received from Italy and Czechoslovakia.

More importantly, the president of the IFMSA, Mr Ian Fraser visited Sudan in April 1967 and was enthusiastically welcomed by the medical students and the then president of the Association, Abdelsalam Gerais. Not surprisingly, Fraser wrote in his annual report '*in the Sudan, I found exceptional hospitality*'. The purpose of this visit is unclear but it is likely that he was exploring the activities and achievements of the Society/Association ahead of approval of its full IFMSA membership.

On the social side, sports activities were popular in the 1960s era and the sports club was one of the most active, alongside the statistics, photography, film show, fine arts and drama clubs, as well as the literary society. The Society had its own football and basketball teams, both of which participated regularly in the inter-faculties tournaments organised by the university student union. In 1964, the Society's football team won the inter-faculties championship for the first time. The basketball team won a similar competition in 1967, beating the faculty of Economics team and in the same year, medical student Imad Omer Zaki, won the Table Tennis Cup.

Most interestingly, there was a Tennis Club where students and doctors played together regularly (**photo 20**). The tennis court was situated on the western side of the faculty premises, an area which is now occupied by the Prof. Daoud Lecture Theatre.

The photography club, making good use of a dedicated photography laboratory in the faculty premises to create their images, aimed to document the students' activities and capture interesting cases in the medical field, while the Club of Fine Arts and Drama as well as the Literary Society, promoted and supported the student's intellectual and creative talents. The latter club was inaugurated in August 1967 supervised by Prof. Morgan, with Society member Ahmed Elsafi, serving as the leading figure. Many sub-societies were formed under the Fine Arts and Drama club umbrella, the most successful being the Music Society which presented over eight musical films and arranged student visits to music institutions, as well as organising a three-month course in the term of 1967-68 in collaboration with the Military Music band. The course was completed by 18 students.

A Statistics team was created in the late 1960s with a duty to participate in both medical and social statistical surveys across the Sudan. . The scope of the team was wide-ranging, involving such fields as:

- A survey of the different regions of the Sudan to establish the normal physiological values of Sudanese individuals.
- A study of economic and social conditions in the community and assessment of health condition in the light of these studies.
- Nutritional surveys for the different regions of the Sudan.

In 1966, the Statistics Team appears to have become well developed as it now had seven student members and four advisory members. Following the presentation of the annual report in August 1966, the following members were elected to hold the offices of the new Statistics Team:

- El Tahir Ali El Tahir - President
- Mohy El Din Abdel Rahman - Secretary
- AbdelRahman El Mahadi - Editor
- Saad Mohd. El Fadil - Business Manager
- Soheir Gahwati (Miss) - member
- Osman Kalafalla - member
- Asim Hamad - member

Advisory members:
- Mr. Ali Kambal
- Dr. Hamad El Neil Ahmed
- Dr. Mustafa Khogali
- Dr. Saad Mohd Ibrahim

By the end of the term 1969-70, the Statistics team had achieved many schemes such as projects for estimating averages of weight, height and growth in Elementary and Intermediate School Students, a questionnaire on smoking and another one for second-year students about life in the faculty.

One of the best loved activities in the 1960s was the Film Show, which took place fortnightly, on Saturdays. The shows were usually organised in co-operation with the British Council, the American Library, and the USA information office. In view of its popularity, a Society member was assigned to lead on this activity as Film Show Director. Mustafa Hammad Kleida was the first to take this role officially in 1967, followed by Salah Abdalla in 1968.

In the early 1960s, the Society launched an annual academic seminar, in which a specific topic was discussed in depth and a summary was published in *Al Hakeem*. The topics discussed in these annual seminars were of great interest and relevance in Sudan. The seminars were well attended by both students and staff, and their recommendations were often submitted to the local authorities for appropriate action. They also received contributions from other allied faculties of the U of K, the Ministry of Health and the World Health Organisation (WHO).

The aims of the seminars were:

- To discuss the chosen subject from all angles in a comprehensive, compact and precise manner.
- To bring to light the social and economic volume of the problem as a whole.
- To question the central measures as applied in the field and find proper measures to assess their success or failure.
- To evaluate the possible advantages of new lines of treatment.
- To submit the appropriate recommendations to the authorities.

By 1969, the following topics had all been dealt with and were published in *Al Hakeem*:

- Infective hepatitis
- Maternity and child welfare in the Sudan
- Development of medical education in Sudan
- Schistosomiasis in the Sudan

- Malnutrition in the Sudan
- Malaria in the Sudan
- Tuberculosis in the Sudan

While the idea of the Debate Group was initiated in 1958, this only became well organised in the 1960s, when bi-annual debate sessions began to be held. As the activity improved, the topics debated became more varied, and it was preferred that they should be non-medical. The debate groups, including the "proposers" and the "opposers", consisted of both students and faculty staff and the atmosphere was usually full of sarcasm and humour. The debate usually concluded with a vote to establish which group succeeded in convincing the audience. Typically, one of the Society members was assigned to head the debate group and run the sessions and occasionally, other faculties would also participate. The first debate session in 1958 was around the question of whether birth control was justifiable or otherwise. Some other interesting topics covered by the Debate Group in its early sessions included:

- The matrimonial state should be entered before the age of twenty.
- Prostitution should be prohibited
- Agriculturalists contribute more to the health and happiness of the people in the Sudan than the doctors.
- Male nursing should be stopped in Sudan.

In addition, the Society organised regular social events, among which were the tea-parties, arranged in honour of the faculty visitors and external examiners, and reception events for new members of the staff and new medical students. The first of these reception events took place in September 1965. In November 1963, the Society took all staff members and students for a social picnic in Wadi Seidna for the first time.

The Society was also visited by delegates of the British Students' Union in August 1965, who were warmly received by the Society President (Ali Elhag, 1965-66), Dr Ali Fadul and Prof. Morgan, showing the Society's links with international bodies, even before joining the IFMSA.

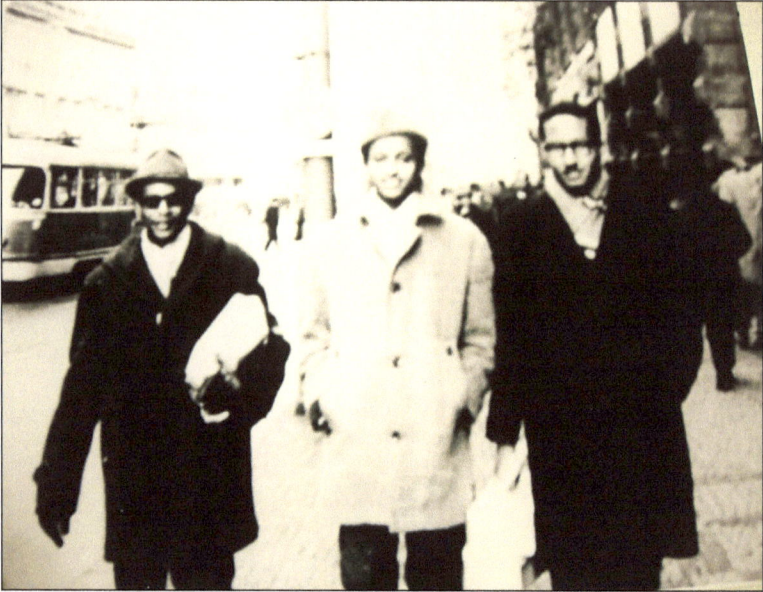

Photo 19: Students' Society members, Mirghani Ahmed Abdelaziz (first from the right) and Mudather Allam (middle) attending the IFMSA meeting in Prague, Czechoslovakia, December 1966/January 1967.

Ahmed Ibrahim Mukhtar was a notable president of the late 1960s who chaired the Association Board from 1969-70 (**photo 21**). Recently, Dr Mukhtar has become the first Sudanese-British man to be appointed to the prestigious role of the High Sheriff of Northamptonshire (2015-16). **Photo 22** shows the cover page of *Al Hakeem* (Issue: 1970). The contents page of that issue displays Mukhtar's letter addressing the Second Annual Congress of the Federation of African Medical Students' Associations (FAMSA). FAMSA was initially proposed by Ugandan students of Makerere

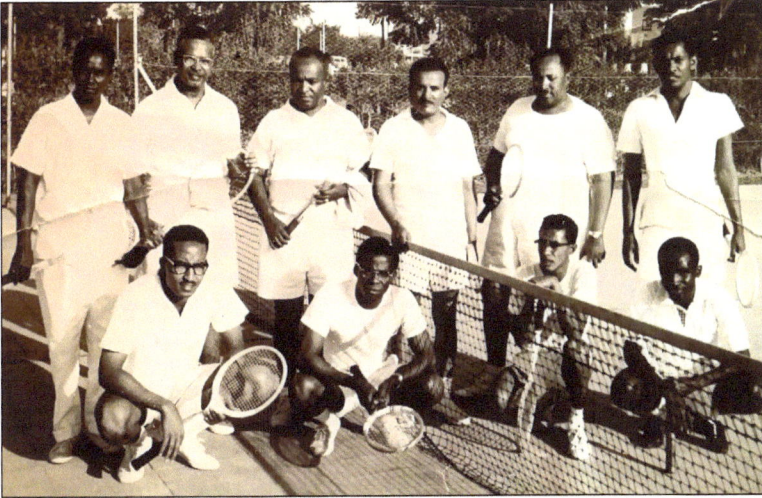

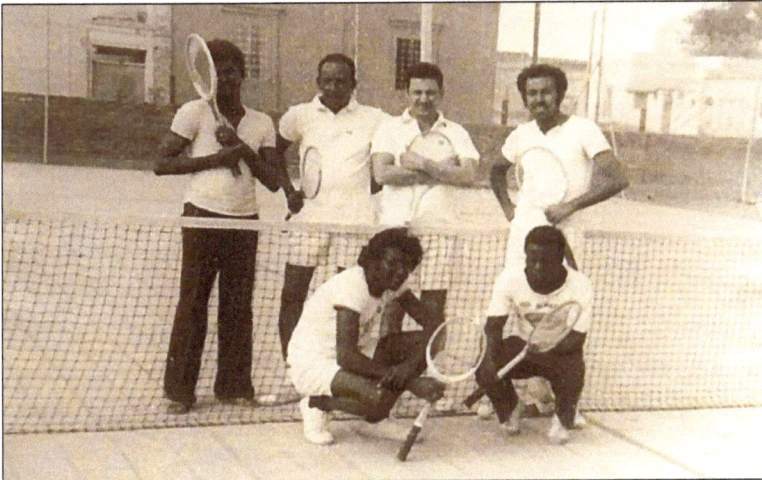

Photos 20: The student-doctor Tennis Club. Top image: Seated from left to right: students Mirghani Ahmed Abdelaziz, Sami (Nigerian Student), Salah Abuelela, Ali M. Abdelsatir. Standing from left to right: Dr. Imam M. Douleb, Dr. Abdelsalam Maghrabi, Dr. Yousif Dafalla Shebaika, Dr. Taha Ahmed Baashar, Dr. Hamadnalla Elamin, student Awad El-Kareem Bashir. Bottom image: Standing from right to left: Tag Elnigoomi, Dr M. Y. Sukkar, Ahmed Osman & Dr. M. Mustafa Kardash.

University in 1965 but was only officially established three years later in September 1968 in Accra, Ghana. The first FAMSA GA was attended by students from Ghana, Nigeria (Lagos), and Zaire and its inauguration was supported by the IFMSA, whose representatives were present at the first FAMSA assembly.

Mukhtar's attendance at the 2nd FAMSA GA in 1969, accompanied by Adil Gamal, the Association Secretary is probably the first documented participation of the Association in regional events outside Sudan. Mukhtar addressed the general assembly of FAMSA and highlighted the history of the Association/Society as well as Khartoum medical school. He gave a comprehensive account of the Society's achievements since its inception and a full report on the objectives and activities enjoyed by the different clubs and sub-societies. He also talked about the vital importance of African educational institutions in fulfilling the expectations of African people in the post-colonial era, as he mentioned:

"We firmly believe that the first demanding duty is the co-operation of all the patriotic African intellects and university students to reflect the real image of the African man giving him his true identity and re-establish confidence in all the splendid past achievements of the African man to try seriously to develop our achievements and publicise them on the universal level.

We feel that we should concentrate and direct all our efforts to Education and the educational institutions. It is very sad that all these institutions in Africa especially our Universities are the last institutions to face the challenges of development and they have failed to plant African nationalism in the African students. This is due to the fact that these foundations up to this day are confused images of the European Educational foundations in their skeletons, in their philosophy."

In his report on the FAMSA annual congress, published in the same edition of *Al Hakeem,* Secretary Adil Gamal discussed its major activities at the event, including a symposium on the role of international organisations in the practice of medicine in Africa, as well as medical film shows. However, it appeared from this report, that FAMSA did not achieve much in its first year, one of the main difficulties, as highlighted in Adil's report, being the lack of funding, because all attempts at fund-raising had proved futile. The assembly also attributed FAMSA's ineffectiveness to the low number of members (only six members out of 20 medical students' associations in Africa at that time).

There was also mention of some informal discussions with African delegates on the issues of Israeli medical students' association membership of IFMSA. Mukhtar and Adil explained why the Sudanese medical students' association would not attend the 18th IFMSA GA which was to be held in Jerusalem. Adil wrote:

"We explained that as students we do not mind Israeli Students being a member of the IFMSA but we do mind and feel strongly about Israeli students running the committee of professional exchange and organising the 18th Annual Conference in occupied Jerusalem, not only because Israelis occupy Arab lands and we are in a state of war but also because the decision violates the IFMSA constitution which states very clearly that All meetings and Congresses should be held in countries where all members can attend. In this case the Arab members cannot attend the conference in Israel even if they want to."

The second annual congress of FAMSA concluded with the following recommendations as indicated in Adil's report:

- The Standing Committee on Publications (Lagos) should publish a "News Letter" containing reports on activities of members of FAMSA and attempt to publish a FAMSA journal, "*Afromedica*".
- The Standing Committee on Professional Exchange (Sudan) was mandated to arrange medical student exchange programmes and to arrange for reduction in travel fares for students.

- The Standing Committee on Health (Zaria) was asked to study the "Health Problems in Africa" as a matter of urgency and to organise blood donation, family planning and health education campaigns.

The author has been unable to determine if Sudan's assignment to establish the African Professional Exchange was achieved in the early 1970s following this FAMSA second annual meeting. However, it does appear that Sudan was also assigned to host the third annual meeting in 1970 but unfortunately, due to poor engagement of the African members, this third meeting had to be postponed.

Omer Ibrahim Aboud, then Secretary General of the Association mentioned in *Al Hakeem* in 1971 that two of the five-member associations, Ghana and Lagos, had notified their inability to attend the congress, which had been planned to take place between the 13th and the 22nd of September 1970. He also mentioned that, since no new applications to attend the congress or to join FAMSA were received, and the attendance was expected to be poor, the congress was deferred to December 1970. Nonetheless, it appears that the meeting never took place.

Interestingly, an Egyptian delegate representing Tanta Medical School arrived in Khartoum in September 1970, having not been aware of the postponement. He was warmly welcomed nonetheless by the Association members in Sudan, and discussions were initiated regarding the possibility of Tanta Medical Students' Association and seven other Egyptian medical students' associations, to join the FAMSA and strengthen the relations with the MSA in Sudan.

It is also unclear if the *Afromedica* journal was ever published in the years following the recommendations of FAMSA's second annual congress. However, Nigerian medical student O.O. Oshin, from Lagos University, who was a member of FAMSA's Standing Committee on Publications (1968-69)wrote an article on the proposal of *Afromedica* which was published in *Al Hakeem* in

1970. In the article, he began by describing the history of scientific journalism and then outlined the anticipated logistic and financial obstacles facing the publication of *Afromedica*.

He concluded:

"In conclusion, the intention to publish an academic journal is reappraised. The central thesis of my paper calls for an awareness among medical students that their association's journal is to be fully fed by articles written by them; it calls for attention of contributors and this association as a whole, through our publications, to the imminent population explosion threatening Africa; it calls for support of introduction of sex education into African schools as means of population control; it calls for adequate funds from the FAMSA Treasury to finance the publication of Afromedica"

Afromedica is currently the official newsletter of FAMSA.

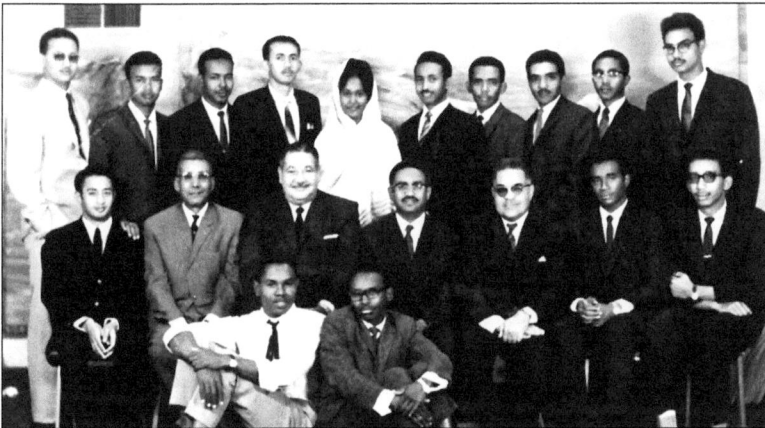

Photo 21: A group picture of the executive board of the Medical Students' Association for the term 1969-70. Seated in the middle row second from the right: President Ahmed Ibrahim Mukhtar. Professor Ahmed Mohamed Elhassan (Faculty Dean 1969-71) is seated right in the middle (middle row). To his left: Prof. M. A. Haseeb. To his right: Prof. Anis Elshamy & Prof. Bakheit M. Omer. Ahmed Elsafi, Editor of Al Hakeem, sits in the front on the right side. Also present in this photo: Maria Satti (standing in the middle).

Contents

1) Editorial
   By M. O. I. Swar

2) Review of history of tuberculosis in the Sudan
   By Dr. Mohyi Eddin Mahdi

3) Human Mycobacteria
   By Hassan Balla

4) Non-human Mycobacteria
   By Khalid Amin Mohd.

5) Bovine tuberculosis in the Sudan
   By A. A. Mustafa

6) B. C. G. works in the Sudan
   By Dr. Mohyi Eddin Mahdi

7) Modern trends in treatment of tuberculosis
   By Dr. El Sir A/Elmagid

8) Scientific Communications
   By Dr. M. Y. Sukkar

9) Kwashiorkor (part 2)
   By Anwar Halwani

10) Mechanism of Sleep
    By Mustafa Nur Elhuda

11) On Afromedica
    By O. O. Oshia

12) Sudan address to 2 nd. annual congress of Famsa
    By Ahmed Ibrahim Mukhtar

13) Report on the 2nd. annual congress of Famsa
    By Adil Jamal

14) News of the Faculty
    Collected by - Adil Yassin & Sharaf El Din A/Rahman

15) قصيدة « غدا تشرق اللقيا »
    مصطفى عبد الله

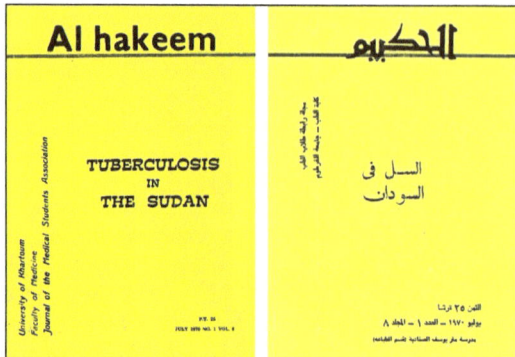

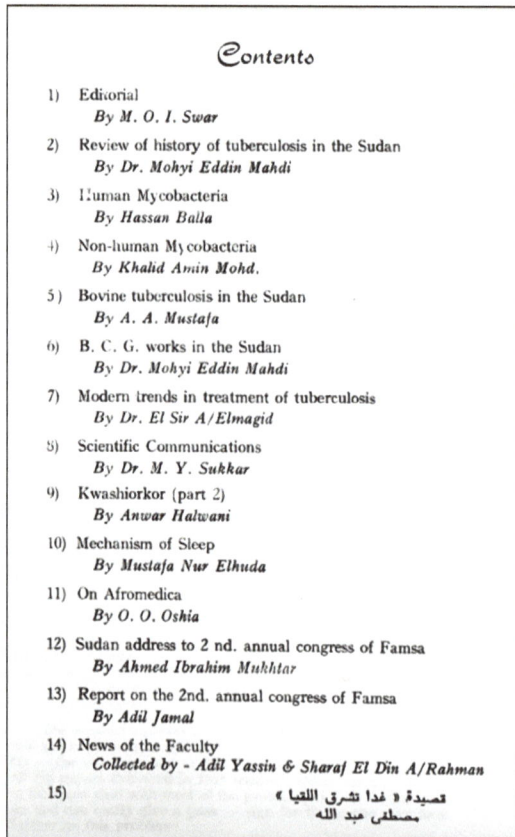

Photo 22: Top: the cover page of Al Hakeem (Issue: 1970). Bottom: the content page of the same issue showing the Association's address to the Second Annual Meeting of FAMSA (Article: 12), given by President Ahmed Ibrahim Mukhtar, 1969-1970.

The author was able to obtain the list of committee members of the Society/Association between 1964 & 1969 from old editions of *Al Hakeem* and they are listed below in a chronological manner:

The term 1964 – 65:
- Osman Mohd Ahmed Taha - President
- Ahmed Said Hamour - Secretary
- El Fatih Abdalla Hamadein - Editor
- Mohd Osman Mekki - Business Manager
- Mohd Ibrahim - Vice-President
- Omer El Farouk El Roufai - member
- Abdel Fatah Abdel Gadir - member
- Hatim Hamour - member

Advisory Members:
- Professor Mansour Ali Haseeb (also Treasurer)
- Professor H.V. Morgan
- Dr. Daoud Mustafa
- Dr. Anis Mohd Ali Elshamy

The term 1965-66:
- Ali El Hag - President
- Riad AbdeLatif Bayoumi - Vice President
- Mirghani Ahmed AbdelAziz - Secretary
- Mustafa Dafaalla Mustafa - Editor
- Abdel Rahman Hag El Khidir - Business Manager
- Hashim Ibrahim Yagi - Advertising Manager
- Abdelsalam Gerais - Distribution and Sales Manager
- Izzat Elias Dawlatly - member
- Hassan Mohd. Ahmed El Faki - member
- Abdelmoneim El Seed - member

Advisory Members:

- Professor Mansour Ali Haseeb (also Treasurer)
- Professor H.V. Morgan
- Dr. Daoud Mustafa
- Dr. Nasreldin Ahmed

The term 1966-67:

- Mirghani Ahmed AbelAziz - President
- Hashim Ibrahim Yagi - Vice President
- Mohamed Sirelkhatim Hashim - Secretary
- Salih Yassin Salih - Editor
- Abdelsalam Gerais - Business Manager
- Wadie Samaan Tadros - Advertising Manager
- Mamoun Hag Ali - Distribution & Sales Manager
- Mudather Alam Ali - member
- Hassan Fadlalla - member
- Hassan Balla - member

Advisory Members:

- Professor Mansour Ali Haseeb (also Treasurer)
- Professor H.V. Morgan
- Dr. Daoud Mustafa
- Dr. Ali Fadul

The term 1967-68:

- Abdel Salam Mohd. Ahmed Gerais - President
- Hassan Fadlalla Ahmed - Vice-president
- Wadie Samaan Tadros - Secretary
- Mamoun Hag Ali - Business manager
- Omer Osman El Khalifa - Editor
- Hassan Balla - Advertising Manager
- Shakir Zein Elabdein - Distribution Manager
- Ahmed El Safi - Assistant Editor

- Soheir Joseph Gahwati - Assistant Secretary – *probably the first female committee member*
- Mustafa Hammad Kleida - Film Show Director

Advisory Members:
- Professor Mansour Ali Haseeb (also Treasurer)
- Professor H.V. Morgan
- Dr. Daoud Mustafa
- Dr. Anis Mohd Ali Elshamy.

The term 1968-69:
- Hassan Fadlalla Ahmed - President
- Ahmed Ibrahim Mukhtar - Vice-President
- Shakir Zein El Abdeen - Secretary
- Samir Ahmed Abbaro - Business Manager
- Ahmed El Safi - Editor (of Al Hakeem)
- Mohd. A. Ali El Sheikh - Advertising Manager
- Ahmed Osman Sirag - Distribution Manager
- Abdel Rahim H. Abu Sibah - Assistant Editor
- Salah Abdalla - Film Show Director
- Mamoun Mohd Ali - Assistant Secretary

Advisory Members:
- Professor Mansour Ali Haseeb
- Professor Daoud Mustafa
- Professor Anis Mohd Ali Elsahmy
- Dr. Makram Girgis.

The 1970s

The Association Leads in Africa

AHMED ELSAFI was one of the prominent presidents of the early 1970s era, being elected head of the executive board for 1970-71. He was an active president and was one of the first members to begin archiving the group's activities. Elsafi was a strong scholar, an effective leader, a talented writer and a skilled artist, who designed the Faculty of Medicine's official logo, still used by the faculty today and also used as the official emblem of the Students' Association. His logo design was selected following a strong competition between medical students, faculty staff members, and students from Graphic Arts. The photo below (**photo 23**) shows the initial draft of the logo.

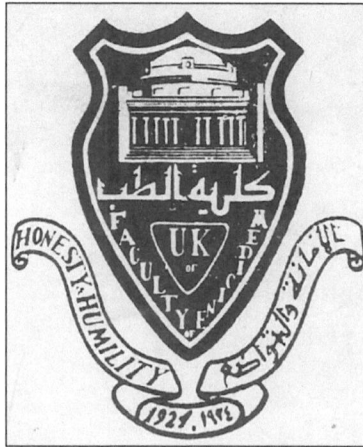

Photo 23: The draft of the logo for the Faculty of Medicine and Students' Association, designed by Ahmed Elsafi. The logo was officially adopted by the faculty in 1966.

Ahmed Elsafi was also on the editorial board of *Al Hakeem* in 1966 (see **photo 13**) and served as Editor-In-Chief from 1968-69. Together with fourth-year students, Yacoub Ibrahim, Amani Hassan Musa, and Anwaar El-Kordofani, Elsafi compiled an *Al Hakeem* bibliography index (1957-67) which was published as a supplement in *Al Hakeem* in October 1968 (No. 2, Volume 7) (**photo 24**). This work was done with the help and guidance of Mr. Gaafar Ibrahim, who was then Assistant Librarian of the faculty of Medicine.

During Elsafi's term as Association President (1970-71), the first archive of *Al Hakeem* magazine was created and in the term 1972-73, a constitutional amendment was made, in order to add a separate, dedicated position of Secretary of *Al Hakeem's* Affairs (Previously Editor), to the executive board. As a result, the magazine now gained widespread recognition, both locally and regionally and even gained official recognition by the WHO. Consequently, it began selling more issues, making *Al Hakeem* one of the Association's main sources of income. A collection of the various editions of *Al Hakeem* is shown in **photo 25.**

Elsafi was succeeded as Editor of *Al Hakeem* by Mohamed Osman Ibrahim Swar (1970-71). Mohamed Swar proposed and implemented the inclusion of more scientific articles written by students; prior to this, most of the scientific articles in the journal were written primarily by faculty staff. Interestingly, previous editors of *Al Hakeem* now began to take on the role of advisory (consultants) for the editorial board and in the early 1970s, Dr Mustafa Khogali, the second editor of *Al Hakeem* in 1958, served as the journal's advisory editor. Among other students who chaired the editorial board of *Al Hakeem* in that era was Mohamed Ali Eltoum (1974), who is currently a well-known endocrinologist and diplomat and has recently served as Sudan's ambassador to Norway.

From the early 1970s onwards, the MSA introduced new roles as the elected committee expanded significantly to include 15 members but it is likely that this constitutional change took place in the term of 1969-70. The main, newly established office in the early 1970s was that of Social Affairs Secretary, while the Financial and Circulation secretaries replaced the Business and Distribution managers respectively. The dedicated position of Film Show Director was abandoned at this point. Each of the seven roles had an assistant in the new structure and now, second-year students were also given a seat on the committee for the first time, with their representative being elected separately by second-year students. As a consequence of these expansions to the Association's board and activities, the advisory committee was also increased to six staff members.

The committee members of the term 1970-71 are listed below:

- Ahmed Elsafi - President
- Abdel Azim Mohd. Kaballo - Vice President.
- Omer Ibrahim Aboud - General Secretary
- Adam Bagadi - Ass. Secretary
- Izz El Din Galal - Financial Secretary
- Mohamed El Mahdi Balla - Ass. Financial Secretary
- Adil A. M. Yassin - Secretary Social Affairs
- Buthina M. Hamza - Ass. Sec. Social Affairs
- M. Osman Ibrahim Swar - Editor
- Hussein Yacoub - Ass. Editor
- Mohd. El Amin Ali - Advertising Manager
- Salma Mohd Suliman - Ass. Advertising Manager
- Ahmed El Suni Salih - Circulation Secretary
- Kamal Mohd. Galal - Ass. Circulation Secretary
- A second-year student.

Advisory Members:
- Prof. Ahmed Mohd. ElHassan
- Prof. Daoud Mustafa
- Prof. Bakhiet Mohd. Omer

- Dr. Mustafa Khogali
- Dr. Abdelhameed Lutfi
- Dr. Nasraldin Ahmed Mahmoud

In this term (1970-71), the first documented Health Education Week was organised and was held between the 24th and 30th of October, 1970. In this week, a series of health education lectures were delivered by medical and pharmacy students at different venues in Khartoum while some talks were also given through Omdurman Radio and Television. At the end of the week, the students left Khartoum in two groups and held outreach health education sessions in Wed-Medani, Fadasi, El-Hasaheisa and El-Kamlin. The whole event was preceded by food and drug appeal campaigns and the collected material was distributed to children in need.

The Health Education Week concluded with a gala night to celebrate its success; jazz music was played and two students, Tigani Adam Hamad and Malik El-Agib, were given presents to acknowledge their pivotal role in making the H.E. Week such a success.

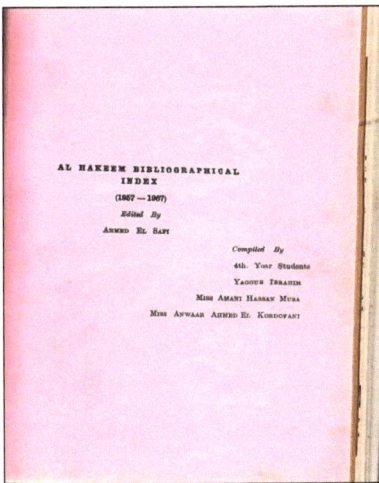

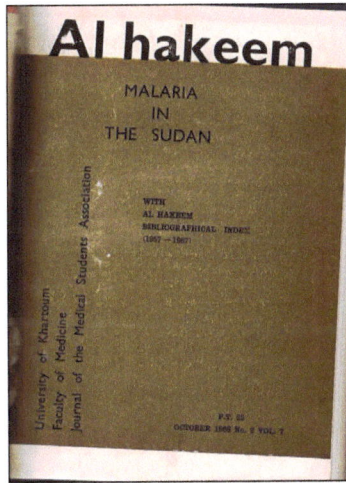

Photo 24: Right: The cover page of Al Hakeem, Oct. 1968 (Editor-in-Chief: Ahmed Elsafi). Left: Al Hakeem Bibliographical Index compiled by Ahmed Elsafi, Yacoub Ibrahim, Amani Hassan Musa and Anwaar El-Kordofani.

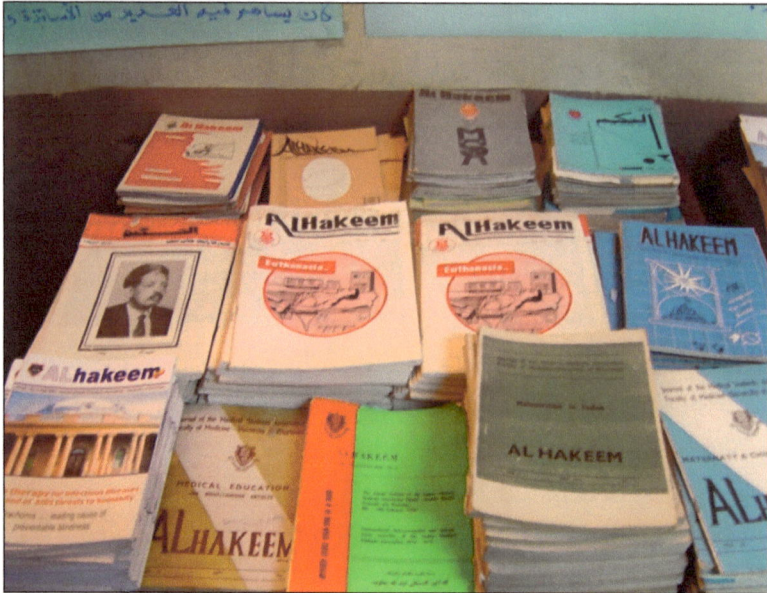

Photo 25: The Archive of Al Hakeem, as displayed at the Golden Jubilee exhibition, 2005.

These different societies remained active in the early 1970s. The Photography club and Society of Fine Arts held exhibitions in October 1970 in which photos, drawings, pictures, and portraits done by students were displayed. Sports activities also continued; in particular, the Association established a Volleyball team, which succeeded in winning the 1970 inter-faculty cup, after defeating the Engineering team in the final match. The year 1970 was in fact, extremely successful from the sports point of view, as the MSA won two other sports competitions in the inter-faculty tournaments, the football and the basketball cups.

Omer Ibrahim Aboud (1971-72), the son of the former president of Sudan, and Abdelrahman Ali (1973-74), were two other famous presidents who chaired the Association in the early 1970s; Omer Aboud and his team can be seen in **photo 26.** In this photo, Mohamed Elmahdi Balla, then secretary of the MSA, who succeeded Aboud as president of the Association, is also present.

Abdelrahman Ali also served as Vice-President (or secretary) in the preceding term (1972-73) and can be seen in **photo 27**, accompanied by Ahmed Abdalla Mohammadani, in Athens in December 1972 where they were attending a meeting of the IFMSA.

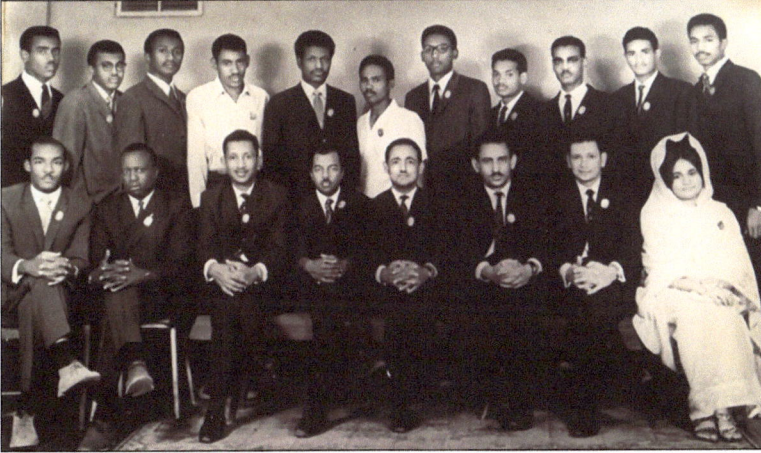

Photo 26: A group photo of the MSA for the term 1971-72. Association President, Omer Aboud, is seated 4th from the left. To his left: Prof. Ali Khogali Ismail (Faculty Dean 1971-74), Dr Abdelhameed Lutfi, Dr. M.Y. Sukkar, Fatima Elsarrag. To his right: Dr. Nasreldin Ahmed, Thomas Gordon, Elhadi Eltayib. Standing from right to left: Mohamed Elmahdi Balla (Secretary of this term and President of the following term, 1972-73), Qurashi M. Ali, Mahgoub Abbashar, Ahmed A. Mohammadani, Aasim Babbo Nimir, Mabyou Mustafa, Abdelghani Fadlallah, Abdalla Abdelkareem, Omer Mustafa Eltinai, Kamal Mohamed Jalal, Moahmed Elhassan Magzoub.

Throughout the early 1970s, the medical students continued to organise community work and field trips. In **photo 28**, students are seen engaging in various activities on a community trip to South Sudan in 1972. Following their return from this trip, the students organised an open exhibition in the faculty, showing the cultural heritage of that part of Sudan which was inaugurated by Abulgasim Mohamed Ibrahim and was later attended by the Sudanese President, Jaafar Nimeri (**photo 29**).

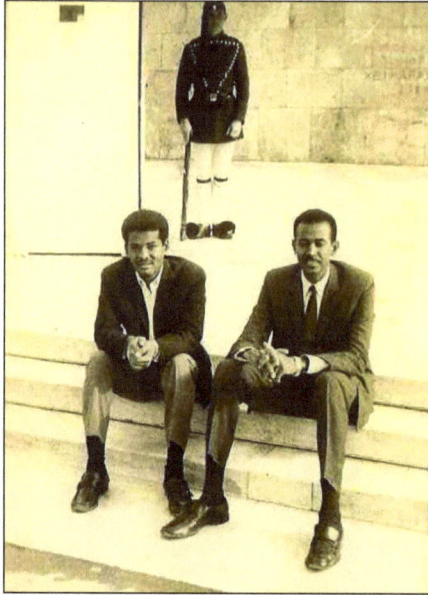

Photo 27: Association members, Abdelrahman Ali (right) and Mohammadani (left) in Athens, Greece, at the IFMSA 1972.

The Association organised a Fine Arts exhibition in the same year in collaboration with the Society of Fine Arts, which had members from all faculties and schools of the University. The exhibition was held in the Examination Hall in the main university campus, and medical student Mustafa Abdalla Salih, and Bashir Omer, a student of the School of Economics, were among the chief organisers (**photo 30**). The event was sponsored by the Youth Minister, Salah Abdelaal, and the Vice Chancellor of U of K, Prof. Mustafa Hassan Ishag.

In 1974, the medical school prepared to celebrate the Golden Jubilee, marking its 50th anniversary. Members of the Association, led by President Abdelrahman Ali and Mahgoub Abbashar, were immensely involved in the organisation for the day and were responsible for the preparation of the various exhibitions. It is claimed that Mahgoub Abbashar wrote a booklet describing the achievements of the medical school over its 50 years. He also published an article on the history of the Faculty in the *Al Hakeem* edition of that year (Vol.9, No.2, 1974).

Unfortunately, due to tensions between the politicised Khartoum University Students' Union (KUSU) and the government of President Nimeri at the time, the event was cancelled. Medical students staged demonstrations, refusing to allow President Nimeri to enter the faculty's premises and preventing him from attending the opening ceremony of the Golden Jubilee. According to Abdelrhaman Ali, as a result of this, the security forces clashed with the protesting students and eventually the medical school was suspended for six months. Abdelrahman Ali and a few other members of the Association were detained by the authorities for 4 months.

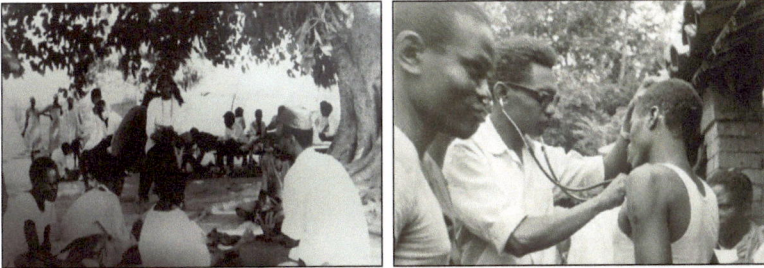

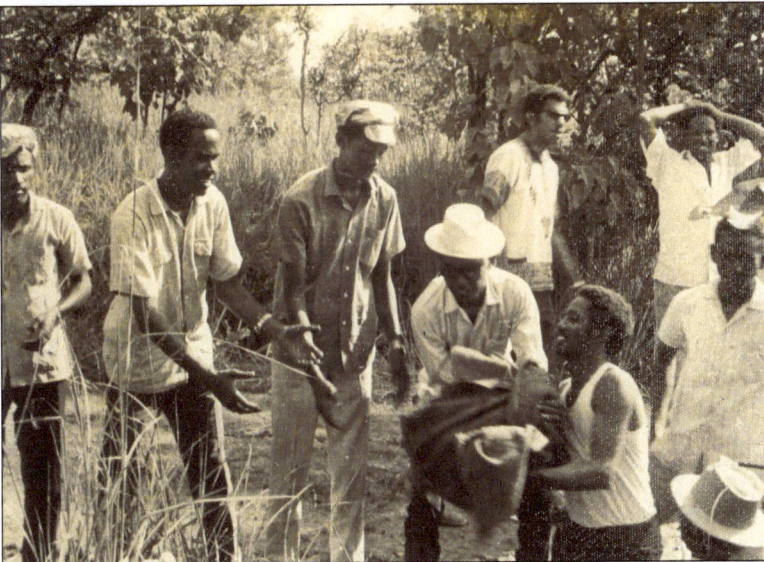

Photo 28: Medical students on a rural trip to South Sudan, 1972.

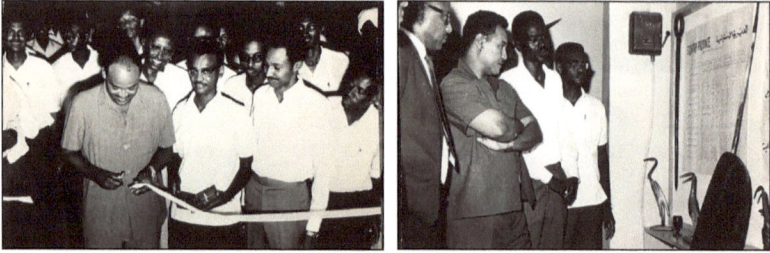

Photo 29: The South Sudan exhibition, 1972. Left-hand image: Abulgasim M. Ibrahim is cutting the exhibition's ribbon. Students Mahgoub Abbashar and Mohamed Elmahdi Balla stand on his left. Dr. Ali Fadul is standing right behind them. Right-hand image: President Nimeri at the exhibition.

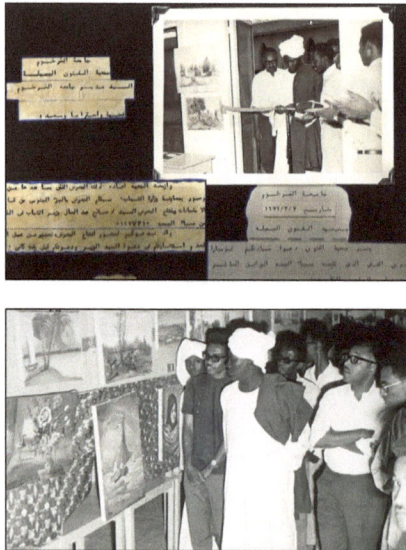

Photo 30: The fine arts exhibition 10/3/1972. Bottom image: from left to right (front): student Mustafa Abdalla M. Salih, Salah Abdelaal (Youth Minister), Prof. Mustafa Hassan Ishag (U of K Vice-Chancellor).

In the mid-1970s, other enthusiastic presidents led the Association, including Tarig Ismail Humaida. One of the achievements of the Medical Students' Association during his term (1976-77), was student engagement in the Middle East. A group picture of the Association board of that term is shown below in **photo 31**.

Tarig Ismail presented a research paper on the medical students' work in developing health services in the Arab world which was presented at the 15th Meeting of the Arab Doctors' Union, held in Khartoum in November 1976 (**photo 32**). The title of his paper, later published in *Al Hakeem*, can be seen in the photo below, alongside a portrait of Tarig Ismail (**photo 33**). Tarig also served as Secretary for Media and General Secretary, in the terms 1973-74 and 1975-76 respectively. The board for the 1975-76 term is displayed below (**photo 34**). The President of that term, who appears seated in the middle of the second row, is Balla Mohamed Elbashir. He had initially served as Vice President when Bakri Osman Saeed was chairing the Association's committee, but later became President, as Bakri was detained by the authorities for political reasons.

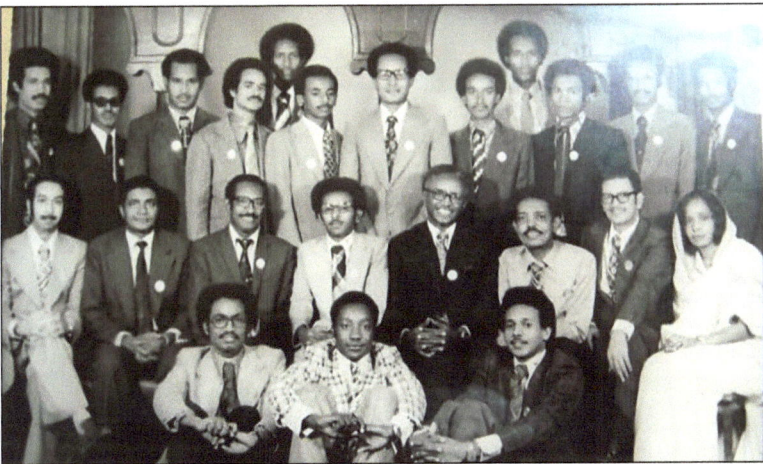

Photo 31: The Executive Board of the Association, 1976-77. President Tarig Ismail Humaida is seated in the middle row (fourth from the left). Faculty Advisors seated in the middle row: Prof. Mohamed Yousif Sukkar (second from the right), Prof. Omer Beleil (third from the right), Prof. Ali Fadul, Faculty Dean (Fourth from the right), Prof. Hashim Erwa (third from the left), Dr. Abdelhamid Sayed Omer (second from the left), & Dr. Mirghani A. Abdelaziz stands in the middle of the back row (sixth from the right).

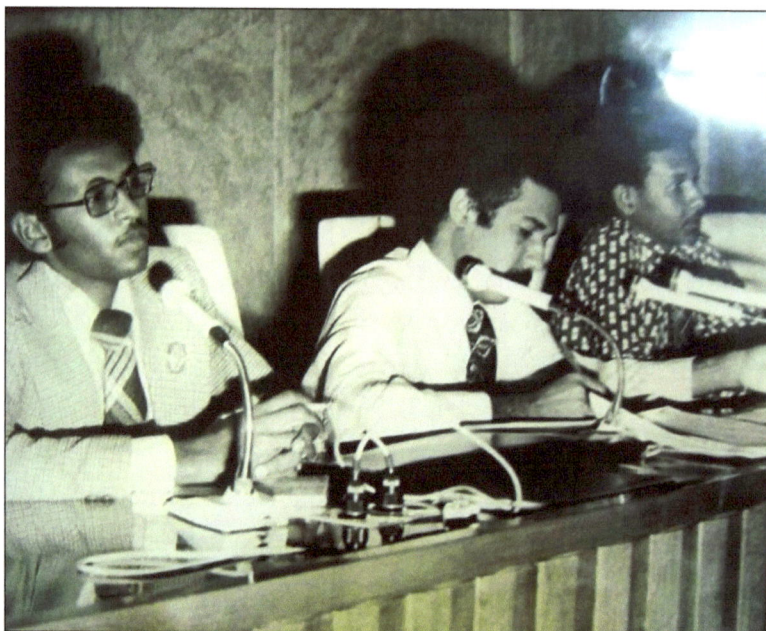

Photo 32: Association President Tarig Ismail 1976-77 (first from the left) at the 15th Meeting of the Arab Doctors' Union, Friendship Hall, Khartoum, Sudan, 1976.

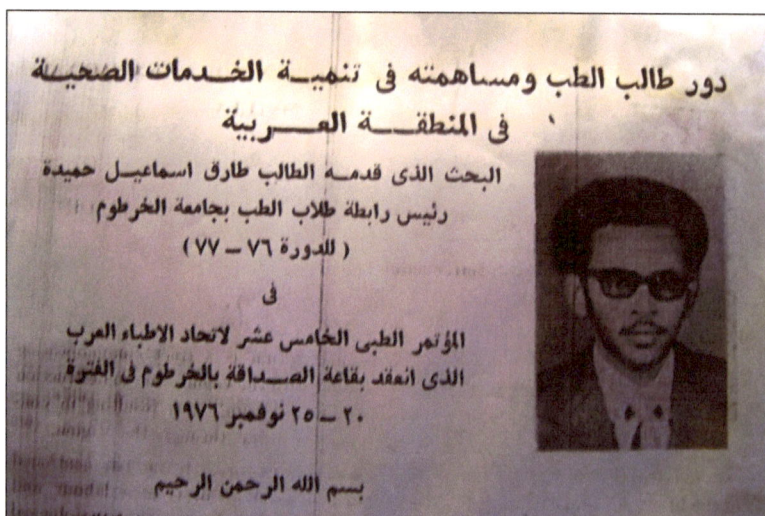

دور طالب الطب ومساهمته فى تنمية الخدمات الصحية
فى المنطقة العربية

البحث الذى قدمه الطالب طارق اسماعيل حميدة
رئيس رابطة طلاب الطب بجامعة الخرطوم
(للدورة ٧٦ – ٧٧)

فى

المؤتمر الطبى الخامس عشر لاتحاد الاطباء العرب
الذى انعقد بقاعة الصداقة بالخرطوم فى الفترة
٢٠ – ٢٥ نوفمبر ١٩٧٦

بسم الله الرحمن الرحيم

Photo 33: The title of the paper presented by Association President Tarig Ismail at the 15th Meeting of the Arab Doctors' Union.

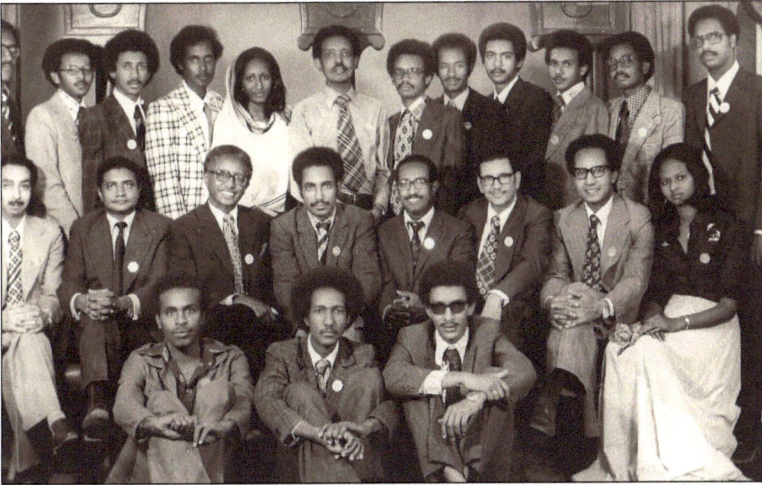

Photo 34: Group picture of the Executive Board, 1975-76. Seated in the middle (fourth from the left) is Balla Mohamed Elbashir, who served initially as the Vice President, and later replaced Bakri Osman Saeed as President. The faculty advisors who appear here are the same as for the term 1976-77 above.

One event organised by the Students' Association in the mid-1970s, was an obituary ceremony in tribute to Professor Mansour Ali Haseeb, which was held at Al-Baghdadi Lecture Hall. In **photos 35** Mustafa Salih, who is currently a prominent professor of Paediatrics, is reciting an elegiac poem with the President of the Association, Bakri Osman Saeed (1975-76), sitting first from the right. The program of the event is also displayed below (in Arabic) (**photo 36**).

It generally appears that MSA Vice-Presidents' typical assignments involved handling external affairs and running the annual seminar, and articles and reports in *Al Hakeem* indicate that Gaafar Mohamed Fageir was deeply involved with FAMSA activities in the early and mid-1970s. During the 1974-75 term, when he was the Association's Vice-President, Fageir headed the MSA's delegation at the Sixth annual meeting of FAMSA in Monrovia,

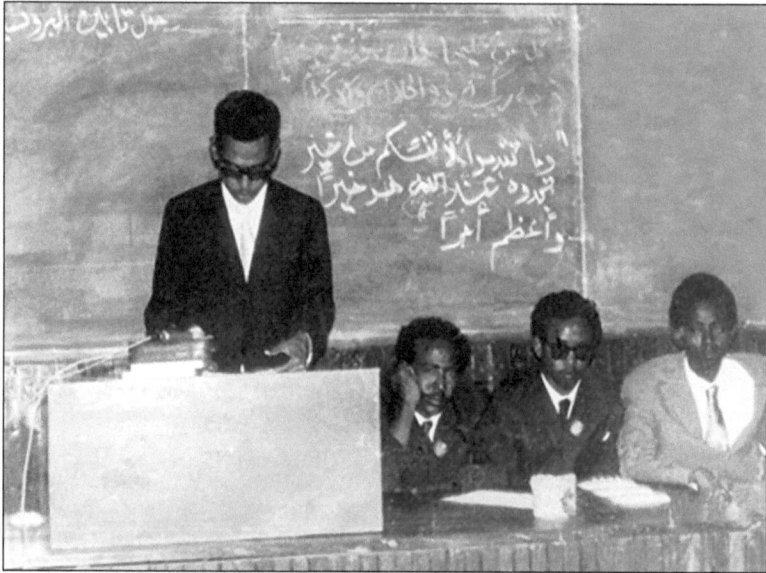

Photo 35: Mustafa Salih reciting an elegiac poem at Prof. Mansoor Ali Haseeb's obituary event in the Al-Baghdadi Lecture Theatre. From the right, seated: Bakri Osman Saeed, Association President (1975-76), Tarig Ismail, Elfatih Mohamed Saeed.

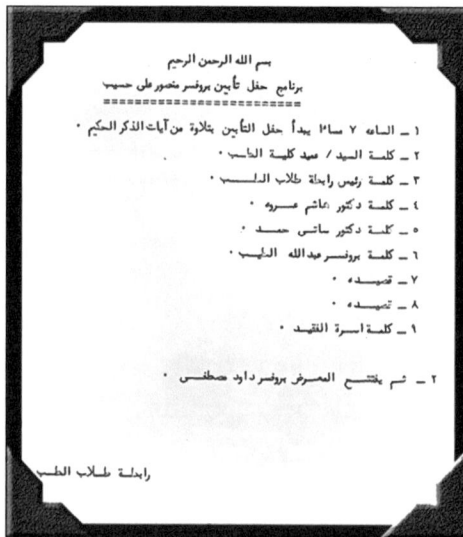

Photo 36: The programme of Prof. Haseeb's obituary ceremony (in Arabic).

Liberia in December 1974, and published a full report (in Arabic) about this conference in *Al Hakeem* in 1978, listing the titles of papers discussed, the activities of the Sudanese delegations and the various workshops held.

In his report, he mentioned that the Sudanese MSA was asked to use its good relations with North African countries, in order to enhance their engagement with FAMSA and encourage their medical students' associations to join FAMSA. The Sudanese MSA was also urged by many Association members to put forward a proposal to host the Seventh Annual Congress of FAMSA. However, Fageir's MSA group felt that the Zambia delegation was very keen to organise the following general assembly of FAMSA, so no proposals were submitted by the Sudanese delegation. Instead, Fageir was nominated and elected as the chairman of FAMSA's Standing Committee on Health (SCOH).

During his term as SCOH chairman, Fageir proposed and supervised many regional health projects. His programme for the year 1975 included the FAMSA Health Corps Volunteers (FHCV) and the FAMSA Drug Appeal projects. The aim of the FHCV was to initiate a permanent corp. to support any recognised African authorities to provide services in circumstances of public medical needs. The FHCV was planned to take place in Southern Sudan in 1976. On the other hand, the Drug Appeal Scheme aimed at raising drugs and materials for the use of medical students' associations in their respective countries, for various purposes including voluntary work and in the student health centres. In the year 1974-75, SCOH planned to organise drug appeals in two African regions, Southern Sudan and Mozambique.

Ahmed Farah Shadoul was elected President of the Association In 1978-79, after serving as Vice-President for the preceding term, and worked tirelessly to re-introduce the Federation of African Medical Students' Association (FAMSA). It is unclear if this body was still active in the late 1970s and Shadoul had to coordinate with other African countries to arrange for the General Assembly of this continental organization. Shadoul, along with his predecessors, Gaafar Mohamed Fageir and Abdelmutaal Bakhiet, talked extensively with colleagues across Africa. In particular, they focused on students from the University of Ibadan, the University of Nairobi, and Makerere University.

In a written statement by Shadoul he mentioned that a preparatory meeting for FAMSA GA was held in April of 1977 in Lagos, and a preliminary committee was formed under his presidency. An Egyptian student, Saif Mukhtar, was the Vice-President of this new committee, which also included members from Nigeria, Tanzania, Benin, Uganda, and Madagascar. Its primary missions were to draft a new constitution for the FAMSA, contact all the African medical schools and prepare for the General Assembly.

The inaugural FAMSA GA was finally held in January of 1978, and in recognition of his pivotal role in forming the Association, Shadoul was elected as President of this African umbrella federation. A Ugandan student took the position of Vice-President, the Secretary came from Nigeria and the office of the secretary was made up of three sub-secretariats; the Secretary General, the Vice Secretary General, and the Financial Officer.

According to Shadoul, Nigeria chose two students to fill the secretary office positions; Dotun O'gunaemi (Secretary - Ibadan Medical College) and Segun Tokedi (Financial Officer - University of Lagos). In that term, the Executive Committee also included members from Tunisia (Faisal Bin Hussein Bey), Kenya (Wamulwa Kebungushi), and Burundi. Sudan's critical role in the reintroduction of FAMSA was formally acknowledged during the general assembly and the first meeting of FAMSA's newly-elected executive committee took place in Cairo, Egypt. A photo of this historic meeting can be seen below (**photo 37**).

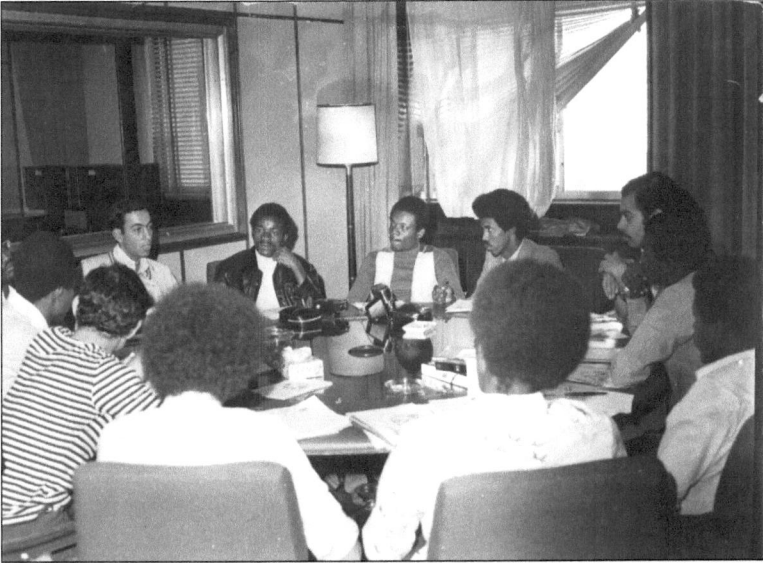

Photo 37: The first meeting of FAMSA's newly-elected executive committee, Cairo, Egypt, 1978.

During his term, Shadoul also initiated discussions with Arab medical student associations in the Middle East; his vision was to create an organization to unite such associations across the Middle East. A preliminary meeting of this new union was held in Khartoum in 1978 which both Egyptian and Tunisian students attended. Due to the fraught political climate, however, most other Arab countries did not send any delegates with students from Syria and Iraq being notably absent. These absences made the inauguration of a unifying body challenging and it is unclear if a far-reaching Arab Medical Students' Association was ever created after that attempt. Locally, Shadoul's executive committee had a significant role in the creation of the Prof. Daoud Mustafa Memorial Lecture Theatre.

In the late 1970s, the Association implemented important structural changes. Female representation became a crucial issue in the medical field and consequently, the post of Deputy Head of Student Social Affairs was usually allocated to a female student. In addition, it was agreed that a student member from South Sudan must be part of the Students' Association Council. The change was made to encourage the participation of underprivileged students from South Sudan—those who were affected by the civil war.

These South Sudanese students were typically granted academic roles, such as Chief Editor of *Al Hakeem*. For instance, Akec Khoc Aciew, who has recently served as the Ambassador of South Sudan in the USA (2012-14), acted as Editor of *Al Hakeem* in 1978. According to Shadoul, while this move did have a political dimension to it, the Students' Association activities at that time were not greatly affected by politics.

Elections took place in February/March, before the beginning of final exams in March and following the faculty's annual "Open Week" celebrations. It appears that the executive team in the late 1970s was increased to 17 members (from 15), with the two additional members coming from the newly established Dental School (1971). Dental students did not yet have a separate student group and at this time, they elected two representatives to the Medical Students' Association committee. The advertisement office also now became the Culture and Advertisement Affairs secretariat, while it seems that the Circulation office was replaced by a dedicated Sports office.

Below is the list of Shadoul's term committee members (1978-79):

- Ahmed Mohammed Farah Shadoul - President (also President of FAMSA)
- Mohammed Nour Ibraheem Nour – Vice President
- Ahmed Hassan Mohammed - Secretary General
- Kamal Mohammed Ahmed Abusin - Ass. Secretary General
- Hassan Ali Mousa - Secretary for Social Affairs
- Faiza Mohammed Ahmed Ass. Secretary for Social Affairs
- Mahmoud Ali Mahmoud - Secretary for Financial Affairs
- Mohammed Elhadi Elamin - Ass. Secretary for Financial Affairs
- Mohammed Salih Ali - Secretary for Cultural and Advertisement Affairs

- Abu-obeida Abdelaal Hamour - Ass. Secretary for Cultural and Advertisement Affairs
- Ronald Ellias - Secretary for *Al Hakeem* Affairs
- Ahmed Yassein - Ass. Secretary for *Al Hakeem* Affairs
- Ammar ELtahir - Secretary for Sports Activities Affairs
- Allam Mahjoup - Ass. Secretary for Sports Activities Affairs
- Omer Mohammed Abdelhaleem - Secretary for Dental Students Affairs
- Salah Barsi - Ass. Secretary for Dental Students Affairs
- Abdelbagi Mohammed Ismail - member: on behalf of Second-Year Medical Students

Photo 38 displays a group picture of the Association's Council, 1978-79 while **Photo 39** displays the board members of the preceding term (1977-78).

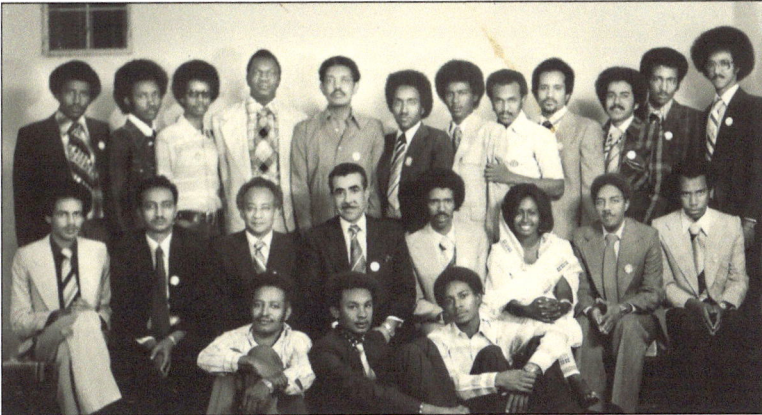

Photo 38: The Association's executive board, 1978-79. President Shadoul is seated in the middle row, fourth from the right. Middle of the front row: Student Ammar Eltahir (currently Faculty Dean, 2009 – present day). Also present: Dr. Omer Aboud (second from the right, middle row), Prof. Elsadig Abdelwahab (third from the left, middle row), Prof. Saad Ahmed Ibrahim (fourth from the left, middle row), and Prof. Beleil (standing in the middle of the back row).

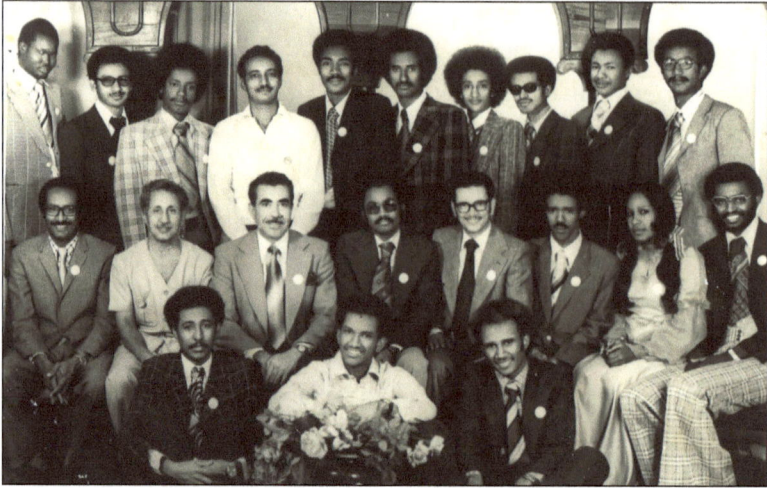

Photo 39: The Association's executive board, 1977-78. President Abdelhaleem Elhidai is seated in the middle row, fourth from the left. Interestingly, four consecutive presidents of the Association are present in this photo. In addition to Abdelhaleem, Shadoul (President 1978-79) is seated third from the right, Aasim Sidahmed (President 1979-80) is standing first from the right and Awad Osman (President 1980-1981) is seated first from the right, front row. Also dental students' representative, Mustafa Osman Ismail (former Advisor to President of Sudan and Minister of Exterior) is standing second from the left while the late Awad Omer Elsammani is standing third from the right.

The Students' Association belonged to the Khartoum University Student Union (KUSU) and its main sources of income were an allocation from the Union, revenue from the canteen, special funding from the faculty dean, revenue from *Al Hakeem*, and funding for medical missions.

In the late 1970s, the Association was very active in the student exchange programme, mainly through the IFMSA. Up to 150 exchange opportunities were available to the students at that time, primarily in European countries, while regional student exchange between African countries was initiated through FAMSA.

The Association's activities during that era were far-ranging and members participated in many extra-curricular sports, cultural activities, and social outings. While student medical missions began in the early 1970s, it was not until the latter part of the decade that these missions became more organised. The Association organised a medical mission to Wed-Medani in 1976, but that mission failed to meet the desired standards and was then followed by a more successful one to El-Obeid, later in the same year. After this, annual medical missions were organised in different parts of Sudan, including Port-Sudan (1977-78) and Kosti (1978-79).

In addition, many sub-societies were active in the 1970s, the most effective of which included the Cinema, Photography, Music & Theatre, and Combating Unhealthy Traditional Practices societies. The Medical Students' Association hosted the first Faculty of Medicine Family Day in the 1978-79 term, which brought together medical students, faculty staff members and their families for an informal gathering, reflecting the close relationships forged between faculty and students during that period. The students also participated regularly in the organisation of the Faculty Week celebration, an event that became popular in the 1970s (**photo 40**). Several social-cultural magazines were also published, many in the form of wall magazines, including *Alwajh Alakhr, Altib* and *Break* magazines.

According to Shadoul, the Association invited many famous Sudanese poets and singers to perform at entertainment nights, which were held in the Faculty on a weekly basis and widely attended by both faculty staff and students. Amongst the singers who performed were Ahmed Almustafa, Abdelkareem Elkabli, Mohamed Mirghani, Wardi and Abuaraki Bakheit. Famous poets Mustafa Sanad, Mohamed Elmekki Ibrahim and Ismaeil Hassan also contributed. The programmes of these nights were often co-presented by the well-known TV presenter Layla Almaghribi.

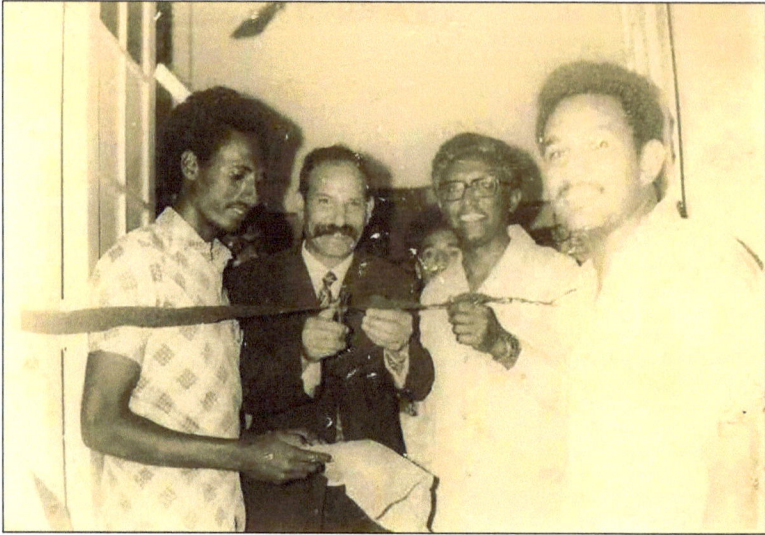

Photo 40: This photo is thought to come from the Faculty Week in the 1970s. Prof. Ali Fadul (Faculty Dean, second from the right) and Prof. Shakir El-Sarrag (third from the right) are cutting the rope of a student exhibition.

The advisory committee (usually six members) of the MSA in the late 1970s included such notable teaching staff as Prof. Saad Ahmed Ibrahim (Faculty Dean 1977-83), Prof. Ali Fadul (Faculty Dean 1975-77), Prof. Mohamed Yousif Sukkar, Prof. Hashim Erwa, Prof. Omer Beleil, and Prof Mustafa Badeh. Previous Association presidents, who later became part of the faculty, were also chosen as advisory committee members, including Mirghani Ahmed Abdelaziz and Omer Aboud.

The 1980s

A Well-Established Organisation Achieving Major Projects

THE FIRST PRESIDENT in the 1980s was Awad Osman (Abu Sheiba), who headed the committee board in 1980-81. Abu Sheiba can be seen in the Association Board group picture below (**Photo 41**), seated third from the left in the middle row. To his right sits the late Prof. Badeh, while Prof. Daoud and Prof. Saad A. Ibrahim are seated on his left.

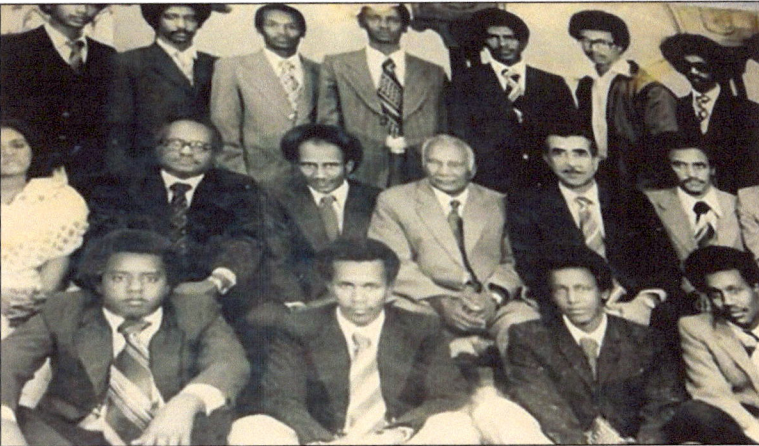

Photo 41: The Executive Board, 1980-81. In the middle, third from the left: Association President Awad Osman (Abu Sheiba). On his right sits Prof. Badeh; on his left, Prof. Daoud Mustafa and Prof. Saad A. Ibrahim.

The same administrative structure remained in place in the 1980s. The President of the newly created Dental Students' Society took one of the two seats allocated to dental students in the

Association board and served as the main Association's Secretary for Dental Students Affairs, elected by dental students only. The second position was elected, together with other members of the executive board, directly from the general assembly of the Association (comprising both medical and dental students). This second representative was usually granted the role of Deputy/ Assistant Secretary for Dental Students Affairs.

The other major change to the election environment was the explicit involvement of political campaigns. It appears that from the early 1980s on, candidates were elected altogether, in groups of 15, with each electoral list being affiliated with a political party. Nonetheless, some of the candidates within these groups still declared themselves as Independent (i.e., having no political party affiliation). During the 1980s, strong competition grew up between the right and left parties in the U of K, for control of the student associations and societies. This competition was a reflection of the general political climate in Sudan at that time, as the disagreement between political parties and the Sudanese President Nimeri, reached its peak.

Perhaps the students soon realised the negative impact of party politics on their associations and representation, as the number of independent candidates on the elected boards began to grow. Initially, the Association was dominated by the *Free Independent* students (between 1980 &1982) but some students began to question the neutrality of this group, claiming it was being infiltrated by members from the right-wing parties (particularly those affiliated with the Muslim Brotherhood). As a result, another group of independent students, known as the *Independent Student Congress*, competed separately in the Association elections, distancing itself from the *Free Independent* group. In the 1982-83 term, only the President, Abdelhadi Abdelgabbar, belonged to the *Free Independent* group while the rest of the board members were affiliated with the *Independent*

Student Congress. The latter group also faced similar accusations, and by the mid-1980s, a third group of independent students called *Al-Mohayideen* (Neutral students) was established.

In 1987-88, the majority of the elected board was formed of these Neutral students (*Al-Mohayideen*). The president of this term was Haydar Giha, who had also served as the Sports Secretary in the preceding term (1986-87), when Nadir Khogali was President of the Association. A photo of the elected board for the term 1986-87 is shown below (**photo 42**). Nadir's term was the last one to be dominated by the *Independent Student Congress.*

The 1970s version of the constitution was still being used in the 1980s when the Association began to have clear and well-defined objectives and the activities of the organisation became well established and more robust. Amongst the Association goals listed in the constitution were the following;

- To develop the intellectual and cultural abilities of students and to guide their skills and experiences towards the building and promotion of society.
- To promote and spread a healthy university spirit among the students and strengthen their relationship with their teachers and other workers in the medical field.
- To promote the academic, social, artistic, and sporting life of students.
- To ensure that students exercise the freedom to express their opinions, within the limits of the constitution, and to reflect the real and vivid picture of the students at home and abroad.

According to Prof. Haydar Giha (President, 1987-88), and Dr Nadir Khogali (personal communication), community work became central to the Students' Association's mission during the 1980s, when many student medical and health education missions

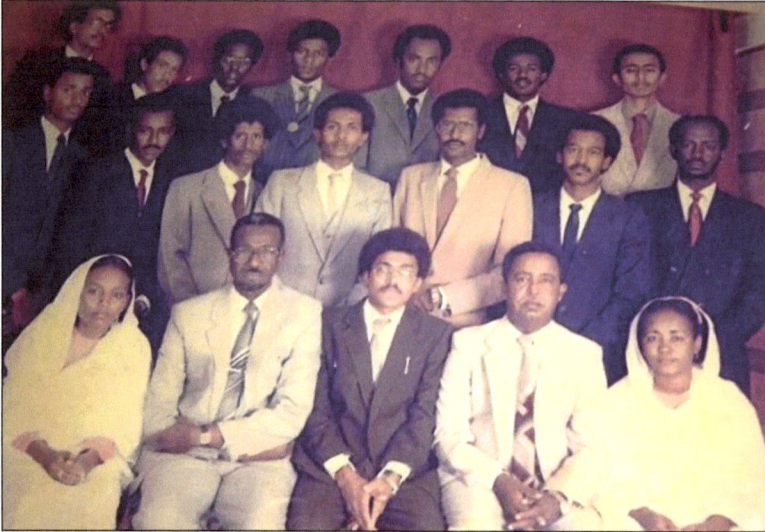

Photo 42: Association Board, 1986-87. President Nadir Khogali is seated in the middle. To his right: Professor Abdelrahman Musa (Faculty Dean, 1983-87); to his left: Prof. Mohamed AH Abdelgalil; Haydar Giha stands in the back row, second from the right. Giha served as the Sports Secretary in this term and became President in the following term (1987-88).

were sent to different parts of the country (**photos 43, 44**). On average, two missions were organised every year, one of which was purely educational. The Association received many dedication certificates from the people of the areas targeted, in appreciation of the students' efforts in improving health care delivery during this time. A collection of these dedication certificates and plaques were displayed at the Golden Jubilee exhibition in 2005 (**photo 45**). The Association also expanded its investment projects and sources of income in this period, as the group hired public transport buses to operate in central Khartoum. The revenues of this project became one of two main sources of income for the Association, along with the canteen revenues. A Commercial Academic & Cultural services Centre was also opened near the canteen and association offices.

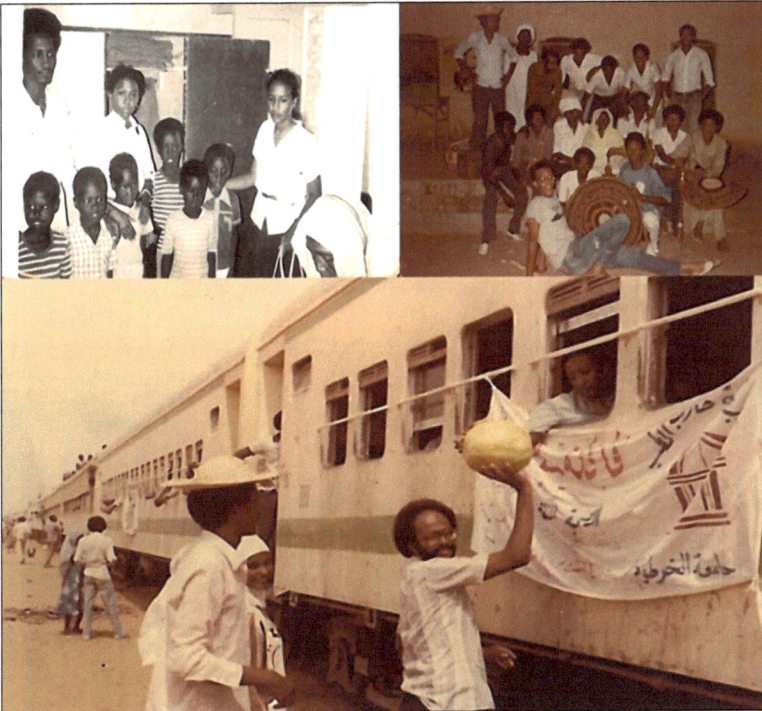

Photo 43: A collection of photos from the various medical missions and educational days organised in the 1980s. The bottom image shows medical students taking the train to Neyala (Western Sudan), Neyala Medical Mission.

Photo 44: The shield of the Association, worn by participants of the medical missions in the mid-1980s. The shield states (in Arabic): Medical Students' Association, Al-Obeid Medical Mission. A depiction of the famous dome of the faculty of medicine building is also printed on the shield and seems to have been used as the Association's official logo at that time.

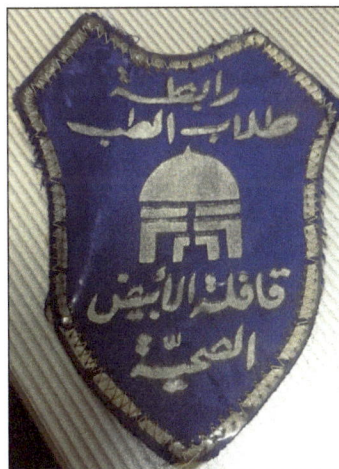

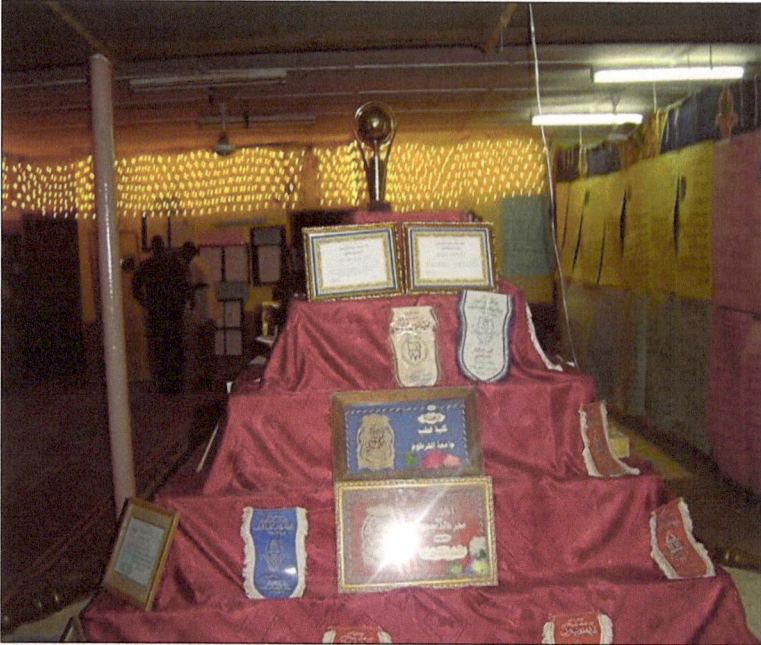

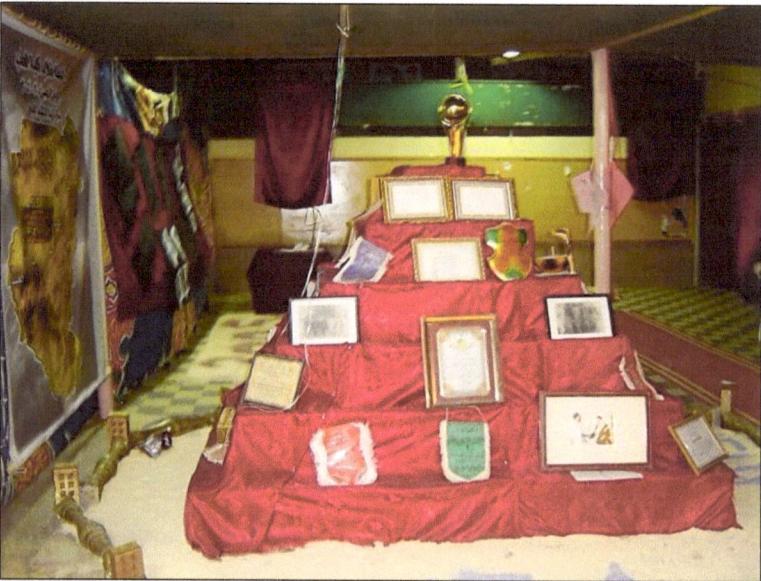

Photo 45: A collection of dedication plaques and certificates awarded by various groups and organisations to the Association from the 1980s onwards. These were displayed at the Golden Jubilee Exhibition, 2005.

The social and cultural sub-societies of the Association became exceptionally active in the 1980s with the number of sub-societies under the supervision of the executive board reached up to 12 by the end of the decade and the beginning of the 1990s. Almoiz Omer Bakheit, a well-known Sudanese-Swedish immunologist, as well as a poet and writer, was the Association's Culture Secretary for 1981-82 and supervised many of these societies.

Almoiz can be seen standing in the back row, second from the right, in the executive committee group photo (**photo 46**). Abdelrahman Almubarak, the Association's President of that term, is seated in the front row between Prof. Saad A. Ibrahim and Dr. Omer Aboud (Association Advisory members).

Other events such as the Faculty Week continued to be celebrated (**photo 47**) and to enhance the social bond between the students, regular entertainment trips were organised by the Association (**photo 48**).

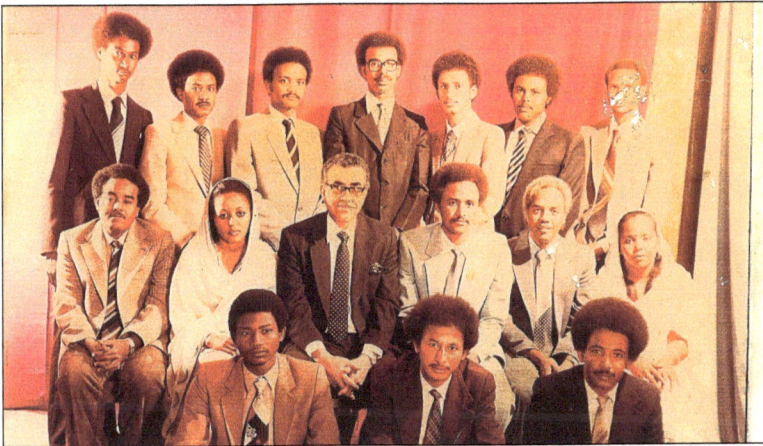

Photo 46: The Executive Board, 1981-82. President Abdelrahman Almubarak is seated third from the right (middle row). To his right: Prof. Saad Ahmed Ibrahim (Faculty Dean) and to his left: Prof. Omer Aboud. Almoiz O. Bakheit (Culture Secretary) stands second from the right. Also standing in the middle is Abdelhadi Abdelgabbar who headed the board in the following term (1982-83).

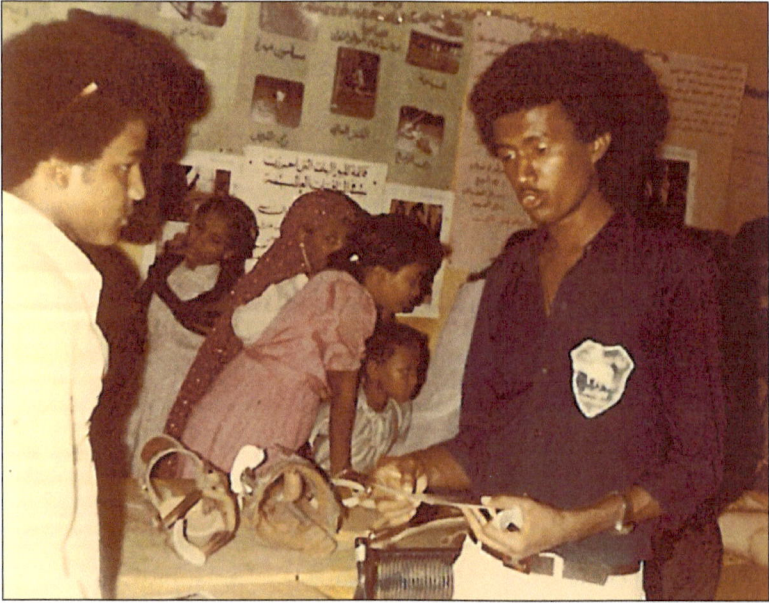

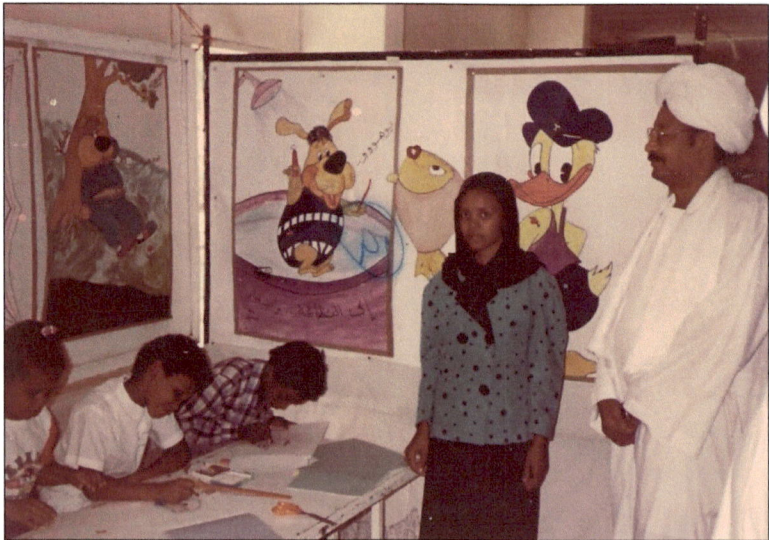

Photo 47: Faculty Week exhibitions. Top image belongs to the 1980s. Bottom image: Faculty Week exhibition in the term 1990-91. The late Dr Mustafa Dafaalla (far right), then Association advisory member, is leading the exhibition's opening tour.

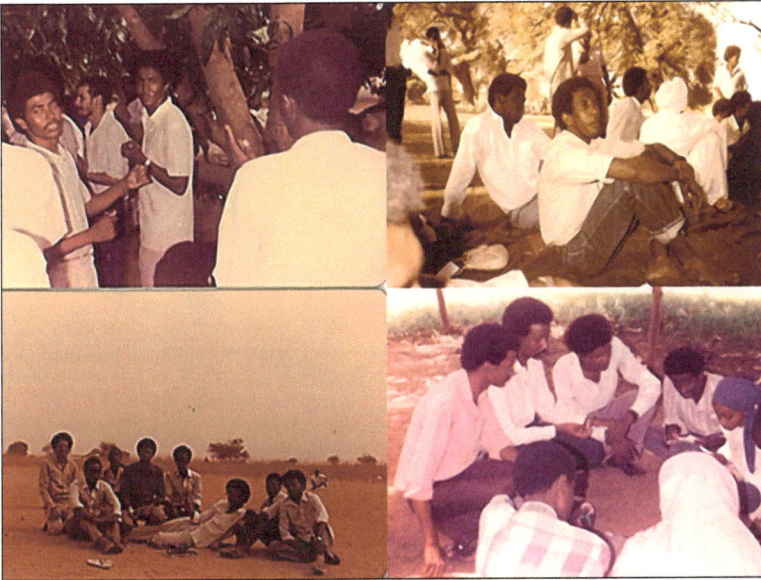

Photo 48: Medical students on entertainment trips organised by the Association in the 1980s.

In the late 1970s to early 1980s, the Association was re-introduced as an umbrella organisation; the Sudan Medical Students' Association (SMSA) and medical students from the newly established Al-Gezira and Juba medical schools were invited to join. Association members from the U of K, in particular Abdelhadi Abdelgabbar, had a major role in establishing the medical students' association of Al-Gezira University and assisted in the drafting of its constitution.

The early 1980s also saw the first documented official representation of Sudanese medical students on the Executive Board of IFMSA. Abdelrahman Almubarak, who was the Association President (1981-82), mentioned (in personal communication) that he attended the IFMSA GA in Australia in 1981 and was elected as Director of the Standing Committee on Population Activities (SCOPA) for the term 1981-82. However, in 1982, the government of President Nimeri suspended the University temporarily for political reasons, and the IFMSA archives show that as a result of this, Almubarak had difficulties in attending the IFMSA meetings and fulfilling his duties of office. During the IFMSA term 1981-82, SCOPA's aims were redefined with a strong need to focus on health affairs and the name of the committee was consequently changed to the Standing Committee on Public Health (SCOPH). Mohyeldin Mohamed Ali chaired this newly formed committee from 1982-83. Mohyeldin was in fact a medical student at Al-Gezira University but nominated by the MSA of University of Khartoum to attend the IFMSA GA in 1982 on behalf of the SMSA. As the SCOPH Director, Moyeldin worked extensively with other members of the IFMSA board to introduce a new community hospital in Wed-Medani (**photo 49 below and opposite**).

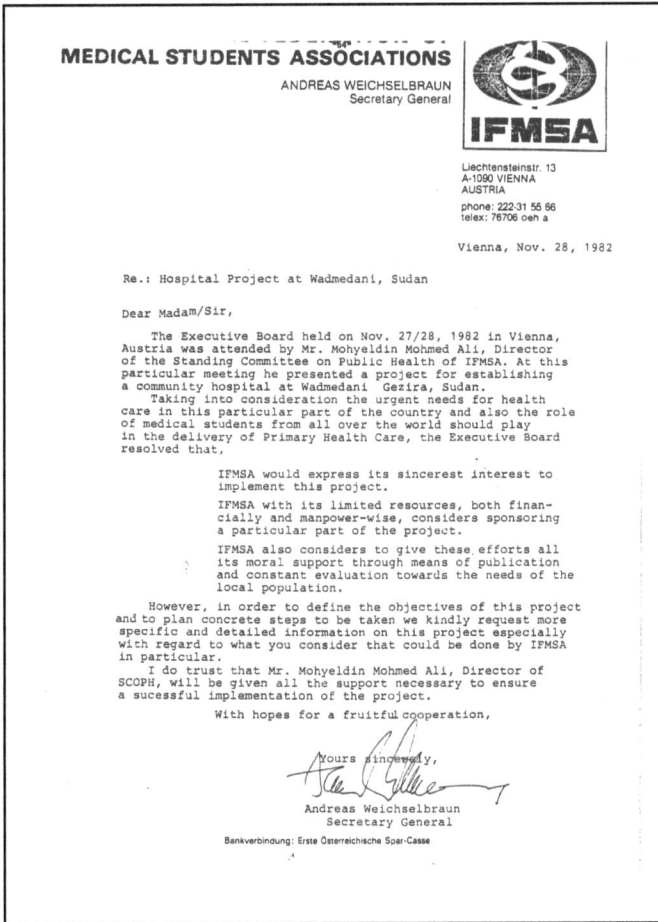

Photo 49: Correspondence between IFMSA Secretary General and Moyeldin Mohamed Ali, SCOPH Director 1982-83, regarding the community hospital project in Wed-Medani (Source: courtesy of IFMSA archives).

In 1984, local collaboration with other medical student associations was taken a step further, when The Medical Students' Association at the University of Khartoum proposed an initiative to include students from the two newly-established medical schools (Al Gezira and Juba), giving them the opportunity to participate in the Students' Exchange Programme through the

SMSA, which continued to be led by students from the MSA of the U of K. By the late 1980s, an agreement was reached between students from all three medical schools, to distribute professional exchange opportunities in the following way; 55% to Khartoum, 30% to Al-Gezira, and 15% to Juba medical students.

In the same year, collaboration between the SMSA and the Kuwaiti Medical Students' Association culminated in successful projects related to refugee aid in Sudan. This success followed the creation of the IFMSA Standing Committee on Refugees (SCOR) in 1984.

Abdelbagi Ahmed, an exceptionally active student, was elected chair of the Association in 1984 and served for three consecutive terms, also acting as Culture and Advertisement secretary in the 1982-83 term and Vice-President in 1983-84.

In personal communication with Dr Abdelbagi, he stated that many major achievements were accomplished in the early 1980s, including, under the leadership of Association President Abdelhadi Abdelgabbar, a complete renovation of the students' canteen and following extensive discussions with the faculty administration, the Association was also successful in building a female student's restroom. This project was initiated by Abdelhadi's team in 1982-83 but was not completed until the following term, headed by Ahmed Abdelrahim Elbashir (1983-84).

According to Abdelbagi, the Vice-President of the Association took on more academic responsibilities at this stage, with the role of *Al Hakeem* editor being confined to supervision of the journal's publication. *Al Hakeem* in turn expanded remarkably and became more popular, gaining wide regional recognition. In 1985, the journal was included by the WHO in the Index Medicus for the Eastern Mediterranean region and the Association also began to publish special editions of *Al Hakeem* in Arabic, mainly aimed at lay readers, focusing on health education topics, to raise their awareness about important public health issues.

The Association was involved in many academic reforms in the early 1980s. Perhaps the major involvement concerned regulation of the controversial process for transferring external medical students (mainly Sudanese students from Egyptian medical schools) to fill student vacancies. The Association had an important role in devising the rules and regulations regarding this process, leading to a reduction in selection bias and more transparency. In addition, the Association members were involved in the issues surrounding the relevance of the second-year exams.

Another major contribution made by the Association in that period was humanitarian aid for refugees migrating from Kordofan to the peripheries of the state of Khartoum, following the declared state of famine and drought in 1984, when the western part of Sudan was heavily stricken with significant drought conditions, resulting in serious food shortages. The Association board, headed by Abdelbagi, worked closely with regional and international non-governmental organisations to provide food and medical assistance in the refugee camps at *Al-Mowaileh* and *Abuzaid*.

A perhaps even larger humanitarian aid campaign was launched by Association members following the major floods in Sudan in 1988. Medical students of University of Khartoum facilitated the provision of food and shelter to the heavily damaged areas and assisted in the delivery of emergency medical aid to people affected by the floods and their hard work in response to that major disaster was commended by the government of Sudan and official authorities.

President Abdelbagi Ahmed can be seen in **photo 50**, accompanied by his team. Unlike other executive board photos, in this one the head of the medical-school bus drivers (Am Ali) was invited to appear. Am Ali was retiring that year and this gesture reflects the close relationship between the students and other faculty staff at that time. Abdelbagi was succeeded by Osama Awad, who led the group from 1985-86 (**photo 51**).

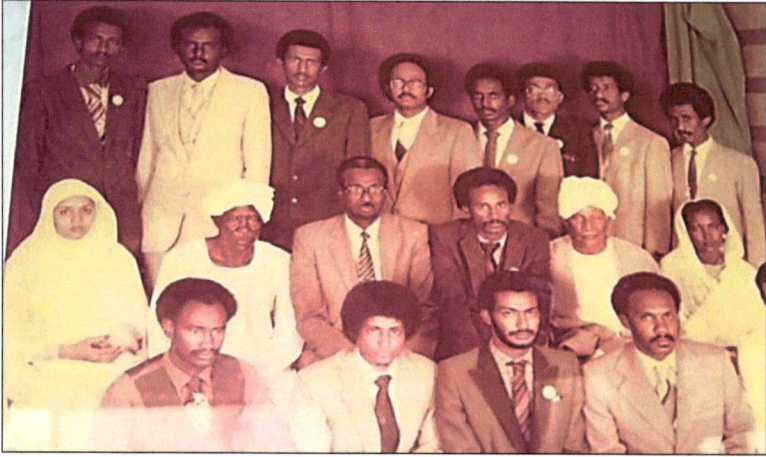

Photo 50: The Executive Board, 1984-85. Seated in the middle third from the right: Abdelbagi Ahmed, Association President. To his right: Prof. Abdelrahman Musa (Faculty Dean) and to his left: Prof. Daoud. Nadir Khogali (then Secretary General) stands third from the right while Am Ali, head of the school bus drivers, is seated in the middle second from the left (wearing traditional Sudanese costume).

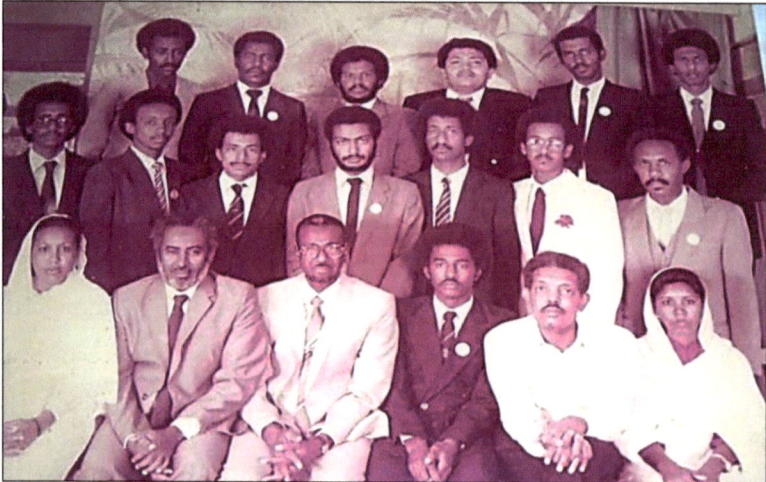

Photo 51: The Executive Board, 1985-86. Seated third from the right: Osama Awad, Association President. To his right: Prof. Abdelrahman Musa (Faculty Dean) and to his left: Prof. Omer Beleil. In this photo Prof. Alsheikh Mahjoub (Microbiologist) is seated second from the left.

As previously mentioned, the late 1980s witnessed the dominance of independent members affiliated with *Almohayideen* group (meaning, "Neutral/Independent"). Hamdeen Hammad Hamdeen, Bahaeldin Abbas, and Essameldin Elamin served as Presidents of the Associations from 1988-90, in succession. **Photo 52** shows the Executive Board of 1988-89, with President Hamdeen sitting in the middle of the front row. In this photo, Bahaeldin Abbas the Secretary of Social Affairs who headed the following term (1989-90), and Essameldin Elamin, the Secretary of Culture who served as president in 1990-91, are also present. The dental students' representative in this board was Hatim Almahdi, who was one of the most active dental students in the late 1980s. He served in two consecutive terms from 1988-90 and then became the president of the Students' Union (KUSU) in 1990-91, the first dental student to hold this position. The group pictures of the two following terms 1989-90 and 1990-91 are shown below in **photo 53** and **photo 54** respectively.

Interestingly, while it seems that medical and dental students had limited participation in the KUSU council throughout the years, their involvement in the Union became more evident in the late 1980s as they managed to lead the council for 3 consecutive terms. In addition to dental student Almahdi, medical students, Hamdi Khalil and Eltigani Elmusharaf were elected presidents of KUSU in the two preceding terms of the Union between 1988 & 90 respectively.

During Essameldin's term (1990-91), the team opened a pharmacy, which enhanced the income of the Association. The project, funded primarily by a grant from King Fahad of Saudi Arabia began in 1989 and the fund approval was facilitated by one of the Faculty's graduates. The pharmacy was officially inaugurated by the end of the term 1990-91, in the presence of the Saudi Ambassador, (**photo 55**). The undersecretary of the Ministry of Health, Dr Khairi Abdelrahman, and the late Prof.

Salih Yassin were also present at the opening ceremony. To date, the pharmacy is still owned and run by the Association.

In the late 1980s, the Association also initiated and supervised the establishment of Prof. Omer Beleil Audio-Visual Library and Surgical Skills Center, as a tribute to the renowned Sudanese transplant surgeon, who made extra-ordinary contributions to Transplant Surgery and Medical Education in Sudan. Beleil also served as the U. of K. Vice-Chancellor (1981-1985), the second medical school graduate to hold this position. The idea was initiated in 1987 but the project was not completed until 1991. Association member Yasir Hassan Sherif with the assistance of Dr Abdelgalil Abdelgader, a Sudanese doctor working in Saudi Arabia, managed to obtain funding for the centre and collected the necessary materials from abroad, including video tapes on various clinical and surgical skills. The centre was built in collaboration with the Education Development Centre (EDC) of the faculty and received great support from faculty members, namely the late Dr Mustafa Dafaalla, Prof. Khalid Yagi and the late Prof. Salih Yassin. The inauguration of the centre was attended by Prof. Mudather Eltingari (Vice-Chancellor of University of Khartoum), the late Prof. Salih Yassin (Faculty Dean), Prof. Ibrahim Ghandour (Head of School of Dentistry) and Essameldin Elamin (Association President) (**photo 56**). Representative members of the family of the late Prof. Omer Beleil (including his brother Osman) were also amongst the attendees.

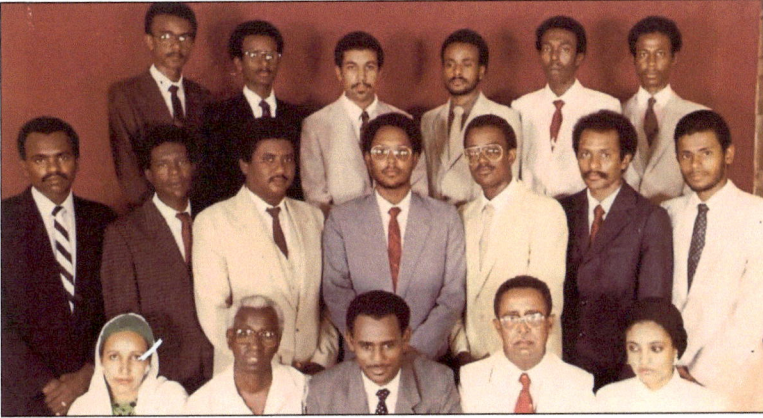

Photo 52: The Executive Board, 1988-89. Seated third from the left: Hamdeen Hammad, Association President. Prof. Mohamed A. Hassan Abdelgalil sits fourth from the left (Faculty Dean, 1987-90); Prof. Khalid Yagi sits second from the left. Standing in the back row third and fourth from the right are Essam Alamin and Bahaeldin Abbas respectively. Hatim Almahdi, Dental Students' representative, is standing third from the right, middle row.

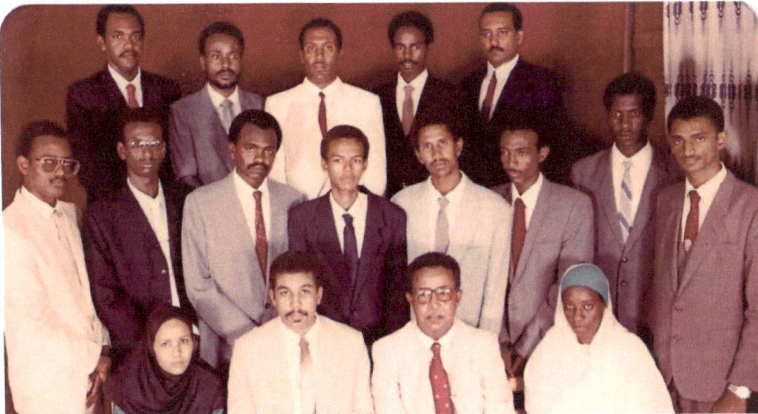

Photo 53: The Executive Board, 1989-90. Seated second from the left: Bahaeldin Abbas, Association President. Prof. Mohamed A. Hassan Abdelgalil sits third from the left (Faculty Dean, 1987-90). Standing in the middle row third from the right: Elsadig Askar (Culture Secretary in this term and Association President 1991-92).

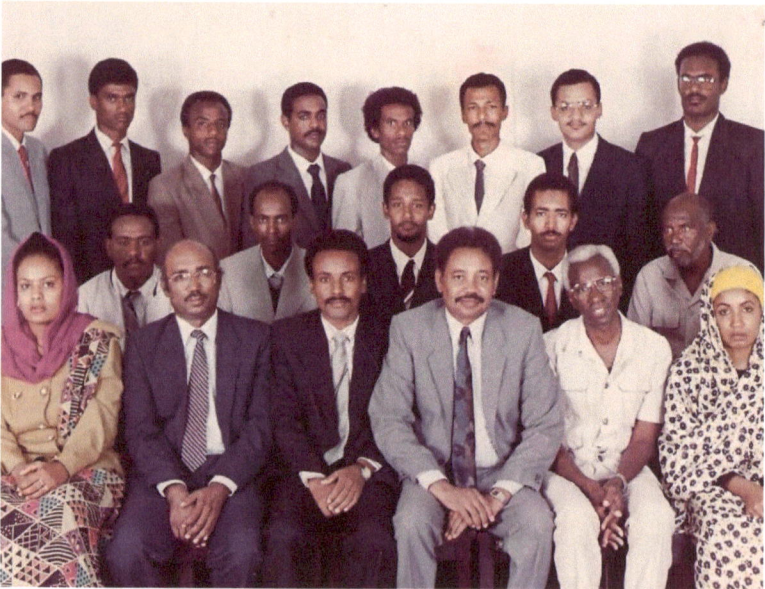

Photo 54: The Executive Board, 1990-91. Seated third from the left: Essameldin Elamin, Association President. To his left sit Prof. Salih Yassin (Faculty Dean, 1990–92) and Prof. Khalid Yagi. To his right: Prof. Suliman Fedail (who became Faculty Dean 1992-94)

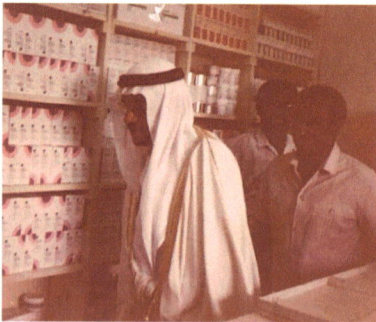

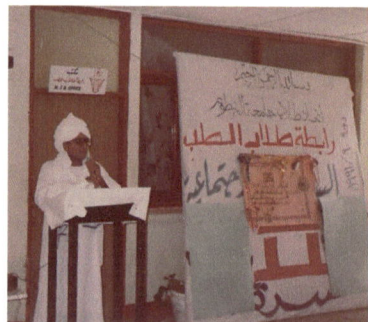

Photo 55: The inauguration of the Association's pharmacy (1990-91). Right-hand image: Dr Khairi Abdelrahman, undersecretary of the Ministry of Health at the inauguration event. Left-hand image: The Saudi ambassador in Sudan visiting the pharmacy.

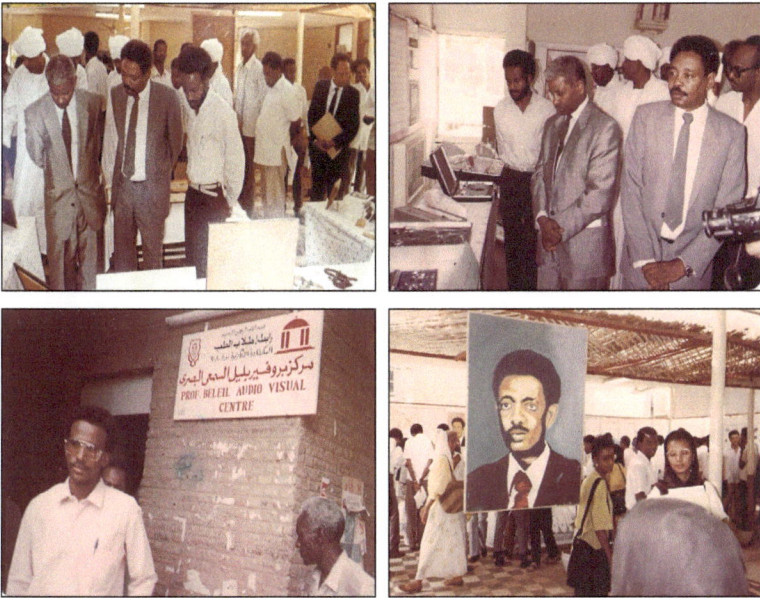

Photo 56: The inauguration of Prof. Beleil Centre in 1991. Right-top image: Standing in front from left to right: Essameldin Elamin (Association President, 1990-91), Prof. Mudather Eltingari (Vice-Chancellor of U of K), and Prof. Salih Yassin (Faculty Dean 1990–92). Right-bottom image: A portrait of Prof. Beleil displayed at the Faculty Week event in the term 1990-91.

The 1990s

The Suspension of the Association

Political instability in the early 1990s resulted in the dissolution of the Khartoum University Student Union (KUSU), which also led to the suspension of the Association. The last term was 1991-92, headed by Elsadig Askar, whose term lasted for less than two months. Nonetheless, the group made major contributions to the IFMSA during that time, as they were deeply involved in humanitarian and community-based activities.

While the Association had officially disbanded by the end of 1991, some activities (particularly the medical missions) were continued by enthusiastic students under the direct supervision of the faculty dean (**photo57**). According to the faculty's book detailing the history of the medical school from 1924-99, the following medical and health educational missions/days were organised by students between 1996 and 1999:

- *Neyala* medical mission - 1996
- *Al-Hilaleya* medical mission - 1996
- *Zalingeh* medical mission - 1997
- *Wad-Hamed* medical mission - 1997
- *Almarabei (North Rabak)* medical mission - 1997
- *Al-Golid* medical mission - 1997
- *Halfa* medical mission - 1998
- *Abu-Jibeha* medical mission- 1998
- *Sinnar* medical mission- 1998

- *Al-Tadamun villages (South Shendi)* medical mission- 1998
- *Um-Eltoyoor (West Al-Damar)* medical mission- 1998
- *Al-Damazin* medical mission - 1999
- *Bara* medical mission - 1999
- *Neyala* medical mission - 1999
- *Al-Bawga* medical mission - 1999
- *Al-Hilaleya* medical mission - 1999
- *Singa* medical mission - 1999

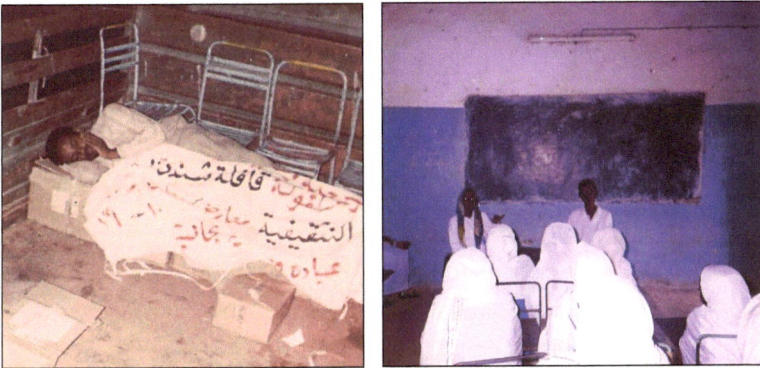

Photo 57: Images from the medical missions organised in the 1990s.

Internationally, the group remained active as Sudanese Medical Students Association (SMSA), which continued to be a member of the IFMSA. Elsadig Askar remained the main point of contact for IFMSA in Sudan for many years.

Khalid Mohamed Eltahir, who also served as the Secretary General of the last legitimate term (1991-92), became the Director of the IFMSA's Standing Committee on Refugees (SCOR) in 1993 and proposed the expansion of the scope of the office to include more work related to peace and war prevention. His proposal was accepted by the IFMSA GA, and the new office was named the Standing Committee on Refugees and Peace (SCORP). Mohammed Abdulgabar Ahmed became Coordinator of this new SCORP in 1994-95.

More importantly, the 1990s saw the implementation of the first and second Sudan Village Concept Projects. The first Sudan Village Concept Project (VCP-1) commenced in 1994 and finished in November 1997; it was proposed by SMSA in Sudan, following its initial success in Ghana in 1988. Sudan VCP-1 was executed in collaboration with the Swedish Medical Students' International Committee (SweMSIC), under the sponsorship and support of The Swedish International Development Agency (SIDA), IFMSA, WHO, and UNICEF. It was conducted in five villages in the El-Gezira state (Umdowina, El Tiboob, Najero, Umjeloud West, and Wad Kerai) and there were also four camps in the project area.

These camps had no names, but were referred to as Camps A, B, C, and D and the project targeted 25,000 inhabitants altogether. Lars Almroth, a medical student from Sweden, acted as the International Coordinator for the project, while locally it was led by University of Khartoum medical students, such as Salah Farooq, Khalid Eltahir, Fadul, and Suhail Ahmed.

The VCPs aimed to achieve self-sustainable improvement of health conditions and general development by following three main principles: integration with the local community, inter-disciplinary cooperation, and international involvement of students. This was achieved by teaming up with local students, working together with villagers, and collaborating to establish general and specific objectives to improve living conditions in the area.

Furthermore, international cooperation allowed international students to participate on a rotating basis, assisting the local students and villagers in achieving the predefined objectives. The project also utilised an inter-sectorial strategy, whereby different sectors (medicine, veterinary, agricultural, dentistry etc) worked together in close coordination. Nearly a hundred local students were involved, and thirty-seven international students from twelve different countries participated in Sudan VCP-1. **Photo 58** shows local and international students standing in front of the VCP sign.

The Sudan VCP-1 was seen as a great success, with most of the specific objectives listed in the original proposal accomplished by the end of the project. Dr Lars Almroth made the following comments on the success of the VCP-1 in his thesis book *Genital Mutilation of Girls in Sudan Community*, which was published in 2005:

"After all activities finished in the autumn of 1997 there were qualitative and quantitative evaluations. These showed that the project managed to achieve many of its goals, but also revealed some shortcomings. One of the main assets for the project was the participating students. They were working for free, out of pure social and professional interest. Totally thirty-six students from twelve countries outside Sudan and more than twice the number of Sudanese students worked with the project. The local and international organising committees consisted only of students. Professional support and guidance needed was attained from the University of Khartoum, WHO, UNICEF, and different NGOs. After this project there was a second SVCP outside El Faw in central Sudan."

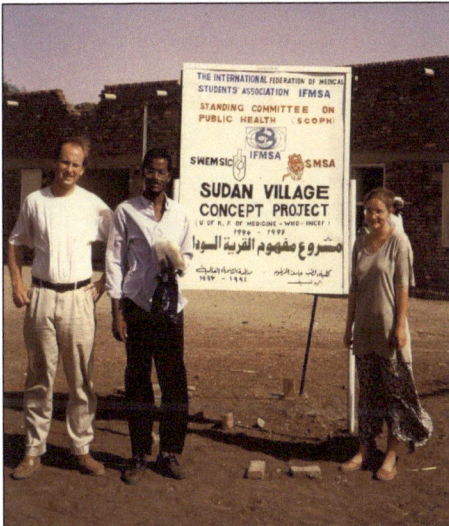

Photo 58: Medical students in front of the Sudan Village Concept Project 1 (VCP-1) project sign, 1994-97. Lars Almroth, Project International Coordinator, stands first from the left. Khalid Mohamed Eltahir, one of the local co-ordinators, stands in the middle.

The success of Sudan VCP-1 led to the introduction of a second project (Sudan VCP-2), which was proposed in 1997 and took place between 1998 and 2000 in five villages in Elrahad Scheme, Elfaw area (**photo 59**). This area, which is part of Al-Ghadarif state, is situated by the Blue Nile, 260km to the south east of Khartoum. The number of international students involved in the second project increased to 50.

The major achievements of the medical sector in Sudan VCP-2 were:

- Carrying out an intensive public health education programme.
- Rehabilitation of three dispensaries.
- Training of 36 health personnel in diarrheal diseases and respiratory tract infections.
- 87% vaccination coverage of the six killer diseases of childhood was achieved.
- Establishment of antenatal clinic at one of the villages.
- Establishment of one labour room with all necessary equipment.

The VCP is considered by IFMSA to be one of their most successful collaborations between medical students and other international organisations. Sudan VCP-2 especially, was often referred to as the biggest developmental work achieved by medical students at that time.

The Sudanese Refugee Project was another humanitarian activity, proposed by the medical students from SMSA in the mid-1990s, which also gained IFMSA recognition. It was based in an Umsagata camp, 100km east of Al-Ghadarif (East Sudan) and the following health services were provided: health education (treatment and prevention of certain diseases), environmental health services (digging pit-latrines), and mother

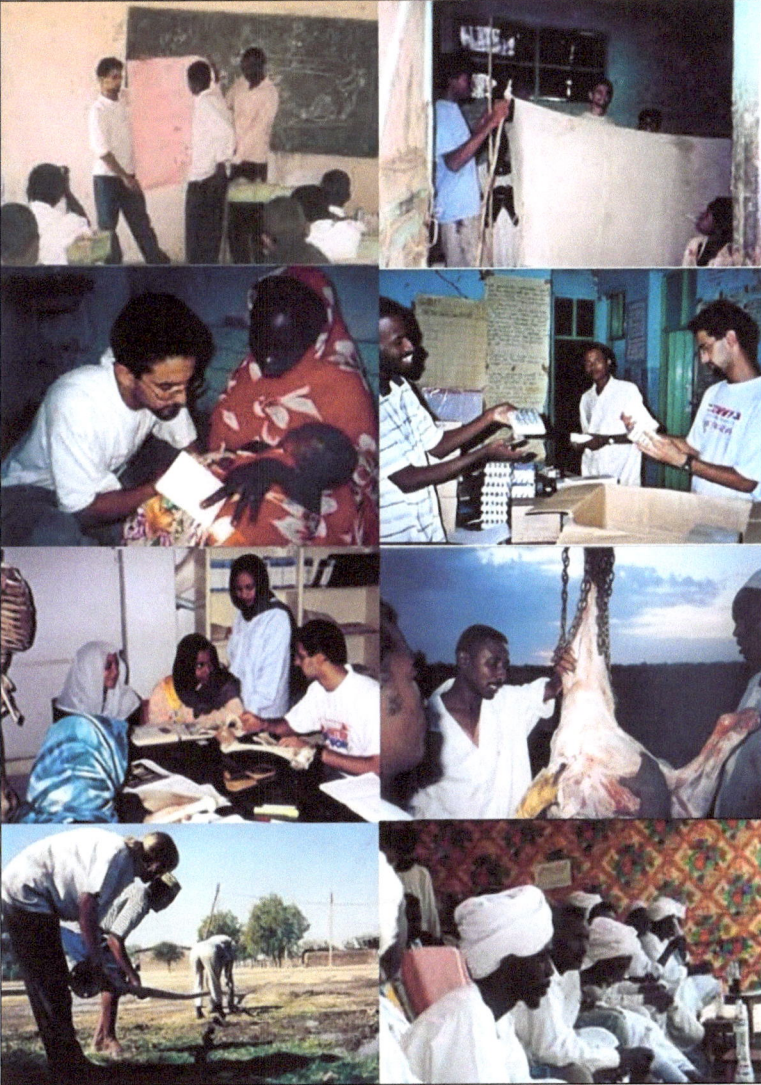

Photo 59: A collection of pictures showing the various activities which took place during the Sudan VCP-2 project. The images reflect the three main principles of the VCP: community (villagers) participation, international students' contribution and inter-sectorial co-operation.

and child healthcare (vaccination, growth monitoring). The project was initiated in 1995, with activity peaking in 1996 and like the VCPs, involved participation from international students. A Sudanese Displaced People Project was also proposed and like VCPs, involved participation from international students. A Sudanese Displaced People Project was also proposed in 1998-99 but it appears that this was terminated following an unsuccessful pilot.

Locally, social and cultural activities continued, in the form of literature and poetry forums and cultural wall magazines, which covered a variety of literature and general knowledge topics. Amongst these popular magazines were; *Afaaq, Lafitat, Abbad Elshams, Itlalah Alsabah,* and *Saloon Altib* (**photo 60**). The poetry and literature forums were also well attended, especially *Al-Shahid, Afaaq* and *the Faculty of Medicine* Forum.

In 1999-2000, the faculty of medicine celebrated its seventy-five-year Diamond Jubilee. Medical students played a significant role in the organisation of this event and fourth-year student Ezzan Saeed Kunna, was extensively involved in the documentation of the history of the medical school. He put together a wonderful piece of work which was released officially as the "Diamond Jubilee book" (**photo 61**) which described the achievements of the faculty of medicine between 1924 & 1999. This project was supervised by the late Professor Eldaw Mukhtar (Faculty Dean 1996-2003) and Professor Al-Zain Karrar, who was then the chair of the EDC.

As part of the Faculty's Diamond Jubilee celebrations, Ezzan also organised and moderated a session titled *Medicine in Old Arabia,* led by such notable speakers as the late, internationally renowned Prof. Abdalla Eltayeb and Professor Abdalaal Abdalla (**photo 62**). Following a wonderful introduction by Ezzan and Prof. Abdelaal, Professor Abdalla Eltayeb then delivered an exciting lecture in his own fascinating style of speaking. He discussed the history of medicine in old Arabia, the contributions made by notable medieval Arab physicians and the overlap between medicine and superstitions in the Arab communities. The lecture was thoroughly enjoyed by the audience.

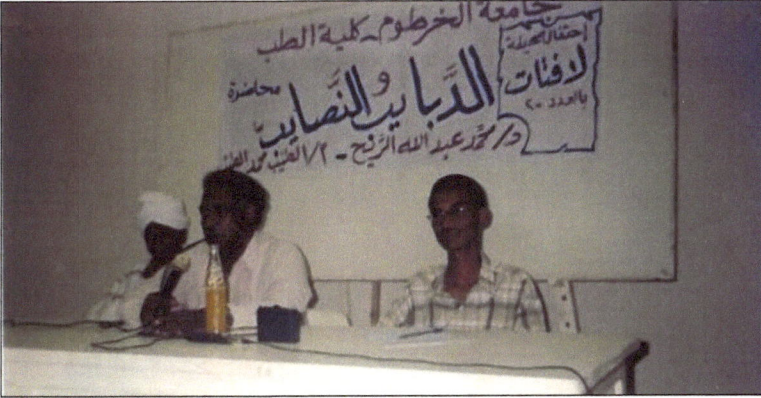

Photo 60: Lafitat magazine celebrating the issuance of its 200ᵗʰ edition at Prof. Daoud Mustafa Lecture Theatre, 2001. Guest speakers: Scientist Dr. Mohamed Abdalla El-Rayah (also known as Hassas Mohamed Hassas) and the famous Sudanese writer and folklorist Eltayeb Mohamed Eltayeb, are seated in the middle and far left respectively.

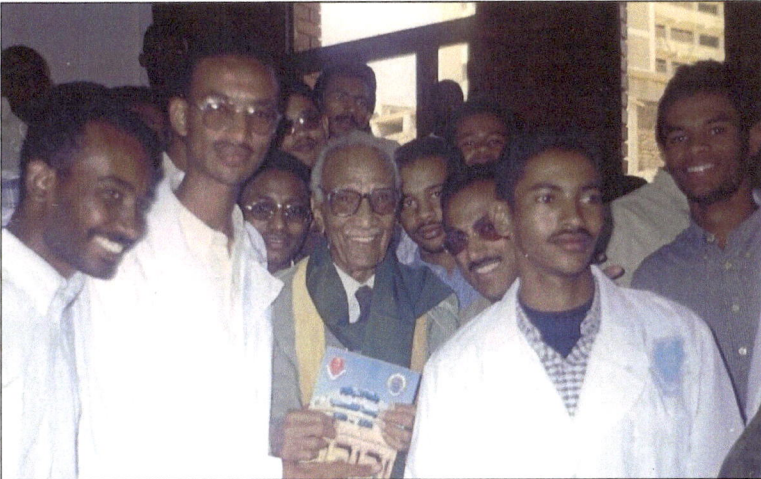

Photo 61: Student Ezzan Saeed Kunna (second from the left) holding his newly released "Diamond Jubilee book" together with the late Prof. Daoud Mustafa (in the middle) at the Faculty's Diamond Jubilee celebrations, 2000. Prof. Daoud, who is considered the father of internal medicine in Sudan, is seen surrounded by dozens of proud medical students.

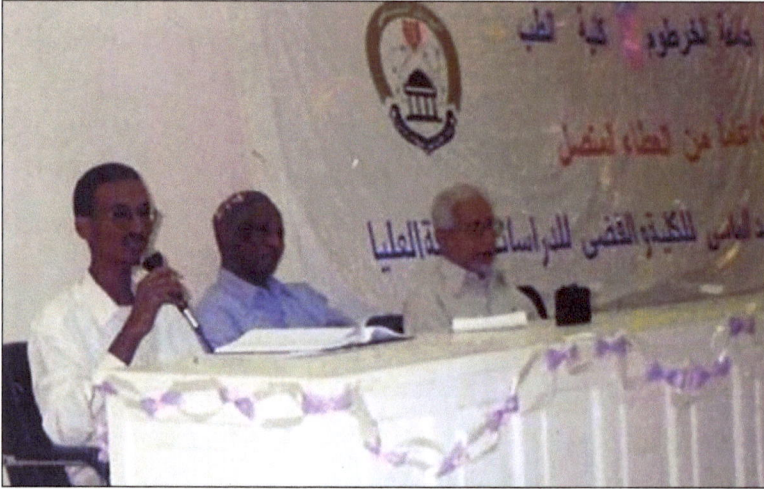

Photo 62: The Medicine in Old Arabia session which was held as part of the Faculty's Diamond Jubilee celebrations, February 2000. From left to right: Student Ezzan Saeed Kunna, the late Prof. Abdalla Eltayeb, Prof. Abdelaal Abdalla.

Another activity that became popular in the 1990s was the second-year Innovations Day (*Youm Alibdaa'*). This was a one-day event in which second-year students (newly arrived at the Medical Sciences Campus) would hold various extra-curricular activities and exhibitions as a showcase of their skills and talents outside medicine. The Innovation Day seems to have replaced the traditional celebration of the 'Faculty Week' which was popular in the 1970s and 1980s and was held under the direct supervision of the faculty dean. This Innovation Day continued as a regular annual event until the official return of the Association and the author has been told that it is still celebrated today. The following photos show some of the activities and exhibitions of the Innovation Day in 2003 (**photo 63**). The author was the head of the organising committee that year.

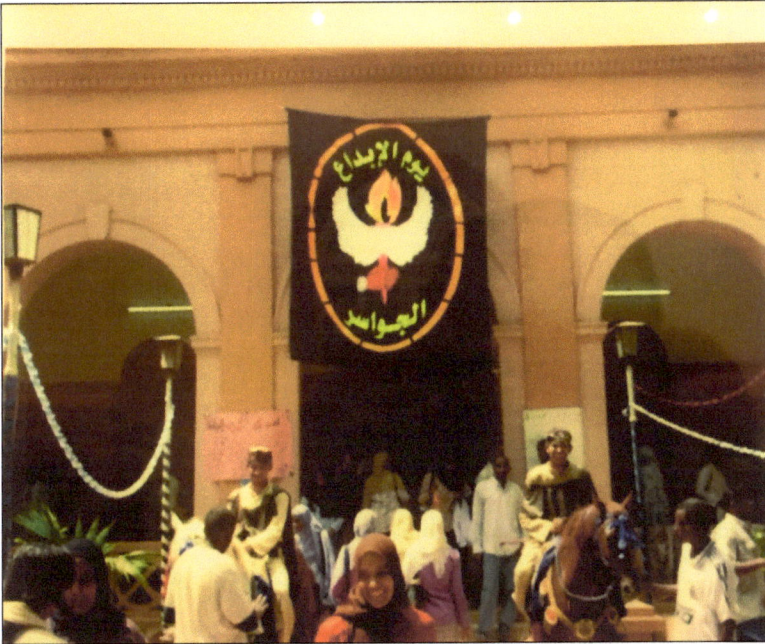

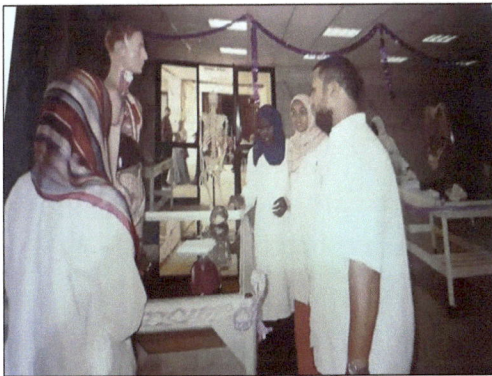

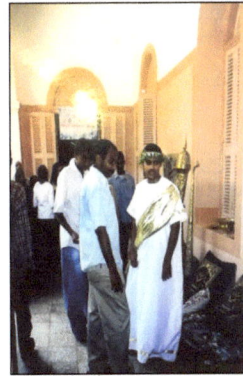

Photo 63: A collection of images from the activities and exhibitions of the second-year Innovation Day, 2003.

The Early 2000s

The Return of the Association

By LATE 1990s, conflicts between students' associations from the different medical schools began to surface and tensions arose following the establishment of over twenty new medical schools in the 1990s, under the government's "Revolution of Higher Education" scheme. These conflicts were primarily a result of competition for control over the Student Exchange Programme. In 2001, medical students' associations from fourteen of the new medical schools decided to form a new umbrella body named initially as SMSA (similar to the name of the original SMSA, which was led by the Medical Students' Association of the University of Khartoum) but it appears that it was later changed to IFMSA-Sudan.

To avoid any threats to the membership of the original SMSA in the IFMSA, the Khartoum medical students led by Mazin Gasim decided to change the name of their SMSA to the Medical Students' International Network – Sudan (MedSIN-Sudan). This change took place in 2003 at the IFMSA March GA in Estonia. The name MedSIN was derived from the name of the umbrella association of medical students in the UK, which is called Medsin-UK.

The Students' Association was officially reinstated in 2003 and was given the name the Khartoum Medical Students' Association (KMSA), referring to the University of Khartoum, in order to avoid confusion with the newly-formed students' associations of other medical schools. A preliminary constitution committee was assembled and its members assigned to write the new constitution for approval by general assembly. The first president following the return of the Association (KMSA) was Elmonzir Bajouri. The main tasks for this new executive committee were limited to setting up and activating the offices and secretariats outlined in the new constitution. This constitution restored the financial resources for the Association and improved students' engagement in the Association's activities.

In **photo 64**, Bajouri can be seen standing on the right-hand side in front of the Golden Jubilee celebration sign in 2005. The author, then student Ahmed MSK Hashim, is standing next to him. Bajouri's team succeeded in drafting the by-laws for the Association's various offices and together with the Finance Secretary, Mazin Ahmed, Bajouri also initiated negotiations with the university administration, which led to the restoration of some of the income sources for the Association (including the canteen). The team also began a process of refurbishment and renovation of the Association office (**photo 65**), which was located next to the canteen.

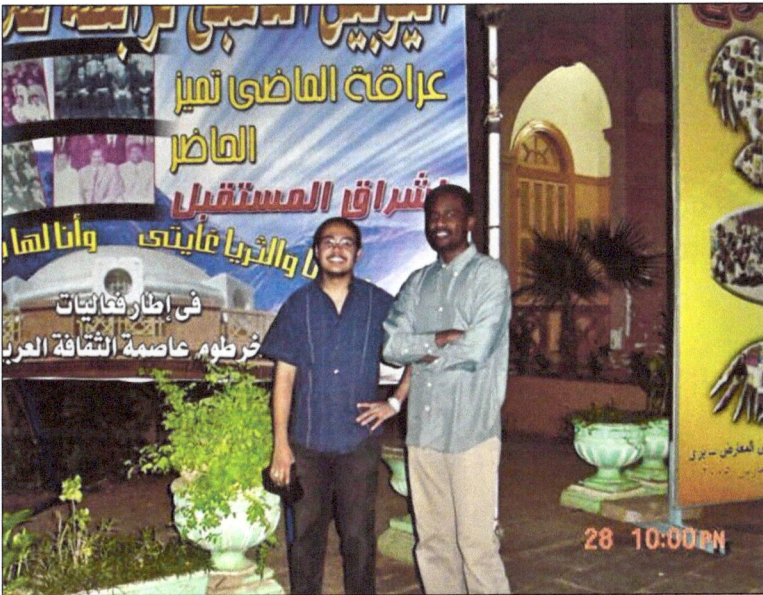

Photo 64: Right: Elmonzir Bajouri, Association President, 2003-04. Left: Ahmed MSK Hashim, author. Both stand in front of the Golden Jubilee sign in the faculty main road.

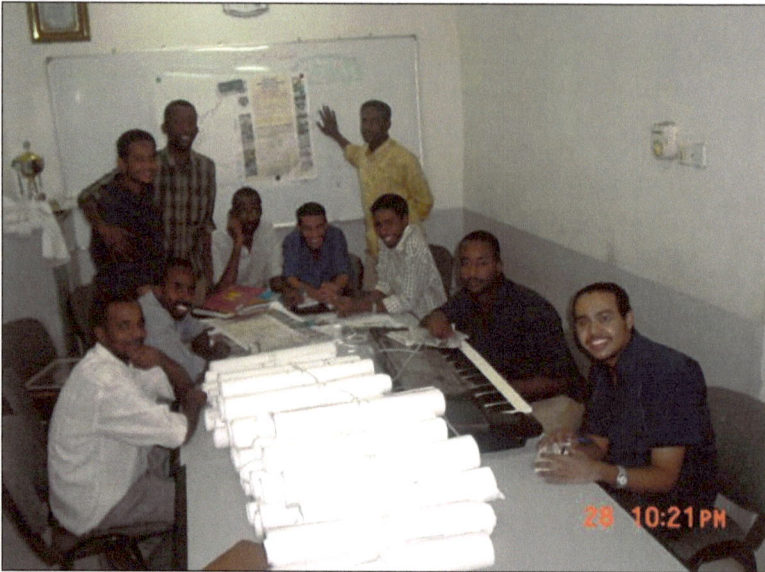

Photo 65: The newly renovated meeting room of the KMSA office. This photo was taken a few days before the Golden Jubilee celebrations and shows student members of the organising committee, preparing for the event.

The new constitution of the Association was proposed and approved in 2003 and the previous 17-member board was replaced by a Council of thirty students which then elected a nine- member Executive Committee. The Council chair had to be a sixth-year student from the final year, while the President of the Executive Board (equivalent to the President of Association) was elected from fifth-year representatives. The Council members were elected using proportional representation, through direct election from each class. Eight members were elected from the second and fifth-years, four members from the third, fourth and sixth-years, while only two students were elected from the first-year.

The new Executive Committee (EC) comprised the following roles:

- President
- Secretary General
- Assistant to Secretary General
- Finance/Treasury Secretary
- Social Affairs and Sports Secretary
- Health Education Secretary
- Academic Secretary
- External Affairs Secretary
- Culture and Media Secretary

2004 - 2005

The Golden Jubilee Term

WHILE BAJOURI'S TERM was successful in restoring the basic administrative infrastructure of the Association, the team of the following term (2004-05) now lacked continuity and experience given the long suspension period in the 1990s was still left with significant challenges. Building teams in the various offices and sub-societies, enhancing student engagement, handling external affairs, and achieving sustainability in funding and income constituted huge obstacles. Nonetheless, the team made remarkable achievements in all areas. The elected Executive Board was led by Ahmed Eltahir Ali (President, 2004-05), while the Council was chaired by Muntasir Ibrahim Osman (Kassala). Ahmed Eltahir is seen in **photo 66** along with other members of the Executive Committee of the Association during the term (2004-05).

This photograph was taken at the University main campus (centre) at the end of an introductory session delivered by the team, to first-year medical students. One of the changes in the new constitution (2004) was the addition of first-year students in the Association's council. Before this, first-year students had no representation in the Association, due to the fact that the first year was traditionally considered a preliminary year, during which students were taught general sciences by the Faculty of Sciences in the main university campus (outside of the medical campus). This meant that logistical difficulties were involved in allowing first-year students to participate in the Association's activities. One of the two year one representatives for the

2004-05 term was Mubashar Abogossi, who served in the Association's board for years and chaired the committee in 2008.

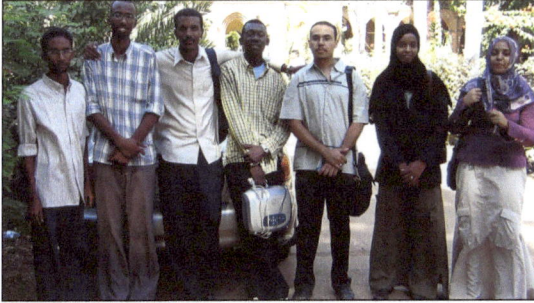

Photo 66: Some members of the Executive Committee, 2004-05. From left to right: Ahmed Eltahir (President), Mutaz Elsadig (Secretary General), Mazin Salah (Academic Secretary), Khalifa Hassan (Assistant to Secretary General), Ahmed Hashim (Heath Education Secretary), Maha Elamin (Secretary of External Affairs), Hiba Abdalla (Culture and Media Secretary).

In terms of academic achievements, the 2004-05 team co-organised the faculty's academic reform conference. In **photo 67**, Mazin Salah, the Academic Secretary, is chairing one of the preliminary sessions with Dr Essam Elkhidir (the chief organiser of the conference). Under Mazin's leadership, a new edition of *Al Hakeem* was published after years of suspension. This edition of the journal is displayed in **photo 68**.

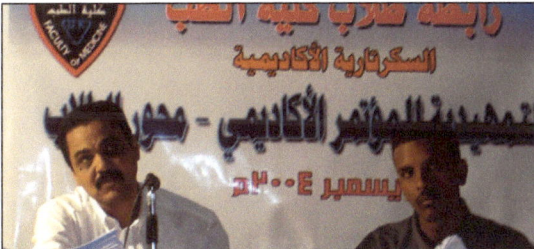

Photo 67: Academic Secretary, Mazin Salah (right) and Dr. Essam Elkhidir (left) chairing the workshop (The Student Axis) that preceded the Academic Reform Conference, December 2004.

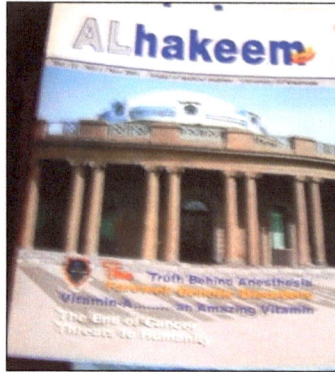

Photo 68: The cover page of *Al Hakeem*, 2004-05.

The secretariat of social affairs and sports, headed by Safaa Elfatih, was one of the most active offices during 2004-05. In a short period, many projects were completed and activities enjoyed. Among those successful projects were the students' Hepatitis B vaccination service, a Ramadan get-together for Iftar, and a cleaning of the faculty premises (**photo 69, 70**). A proposal to refurbish the students' boards was devised and discussed with the faculty's administration, but it faced many implementation challenges. However, the office assisted many students who were facing difficulties with tuition fees and studying expenses. Sports tournaments in football, table tennis, and pool were also organised (**photo 71**).

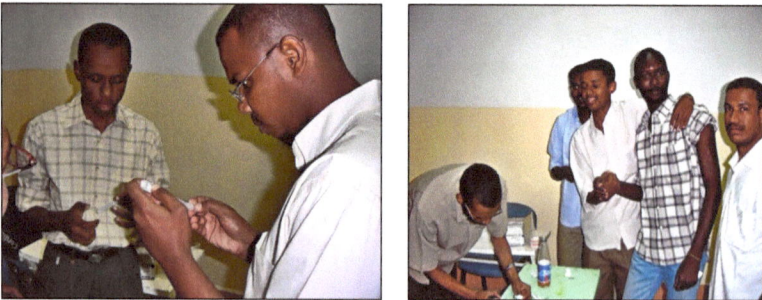

Photo 69: The Hepatitis B vaccination service for medical students, organised by the Social Secretariat, 2004-05.

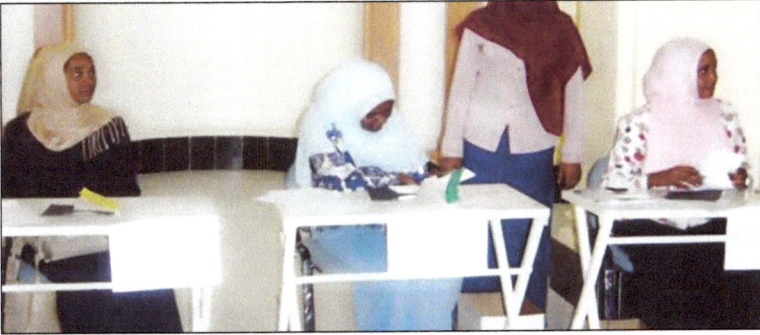

Photo 69a: The Hepatitis B vaccination service for medical students, organised by the Social Secretariat, 2004-05.

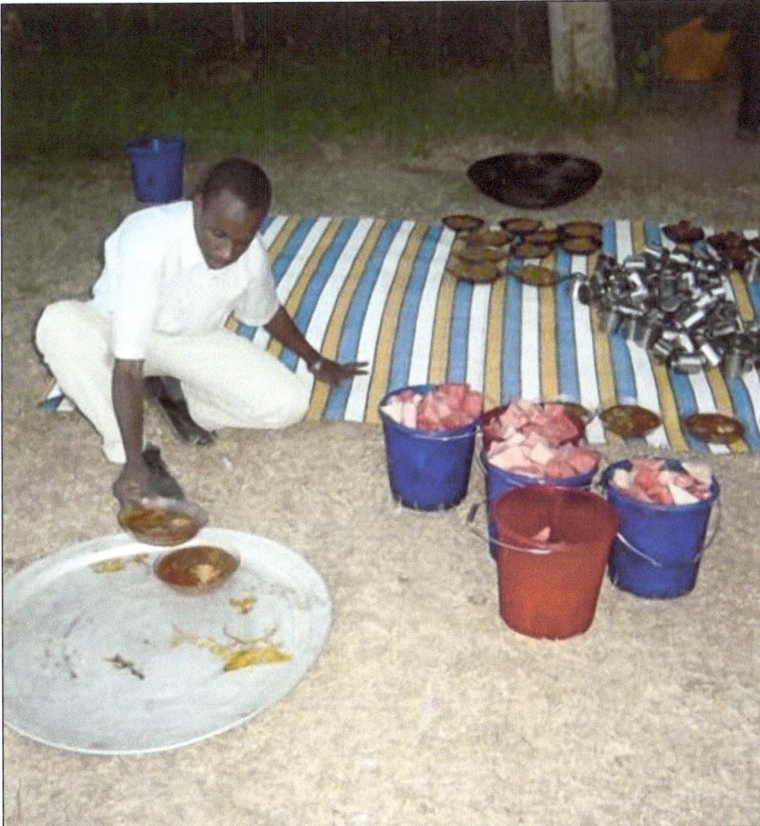

Photo 70: Student Ayman Eltayeb (member of the Association Council) serving food in the Iftar, 2004.

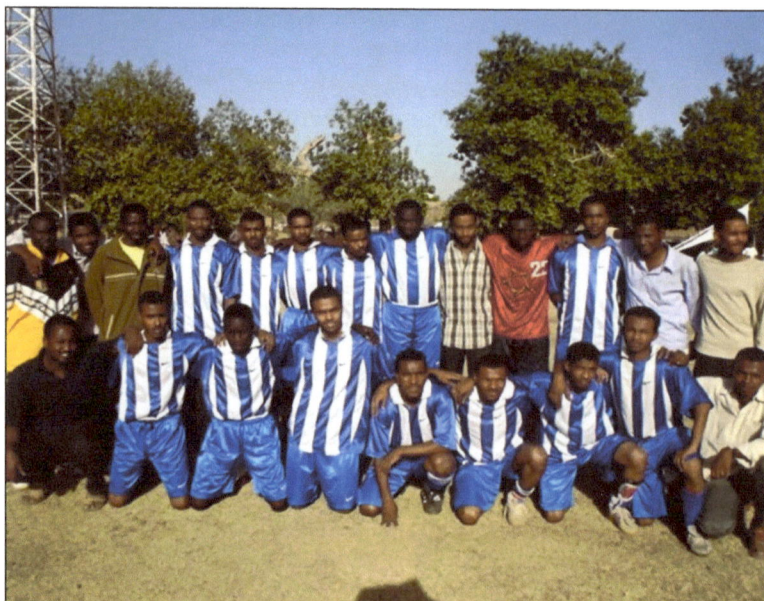

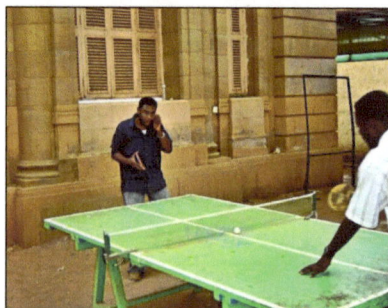

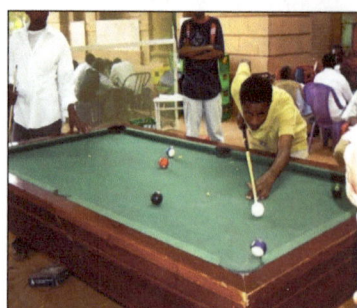

Photo 71: Activities organised by the Sports Section of the Social Secretariat (2004 – 05). On top: The Faculty of Medicine football team.

The newly established Secretariat of Health Education organised many medical missions and open educational-medical days (**photo 72**) and at least seven student-led medical missions were sent to different parts of the country between 2004 and 2005 alone. The author, serving as the Secretary of Health Education, delivered a presentation on medical missions at the IFMSA GA in Antalya-Turkey in 2005 and the Association's Sudan Medical Missions (SMM) were officially accepted by the IFMSA as a locally endorsed project (**photo 73**).

The vision for the future was to allow international students to participate in the medical missions in Sudan, through a formal exchange process but this idea has only been taken a step further recently, when the Association introduced the Sudan Tropical Exchange Project.

Under the supervision of the Secretary of Health Education, many educational days were held within the faculty premises, including a World No Tobacco Day, an HIV day, and a debate session on female circumcision (**photos 74, 75**). The term had also witnessed the creation of sub-societies on Malaria and TB, led by Azmi Omara and Mohamed Abdelwahab respectively. These sub-societies worked in close collaboration with the anti-Malaria and TB National Programmes, affiliated with the Ministry of Health.

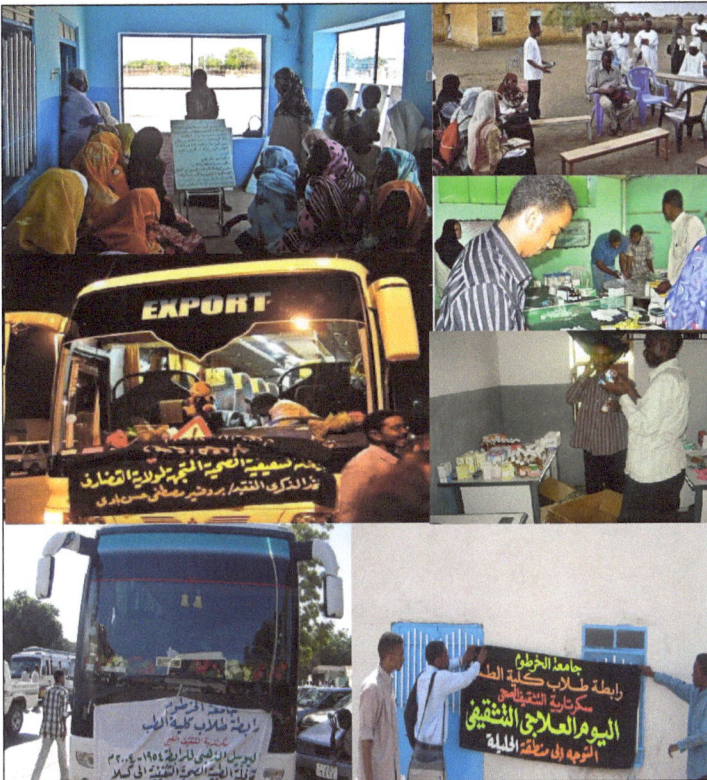

Photo 72: A collection of pictures from the various health education days and medical missions organised in 2004-05.

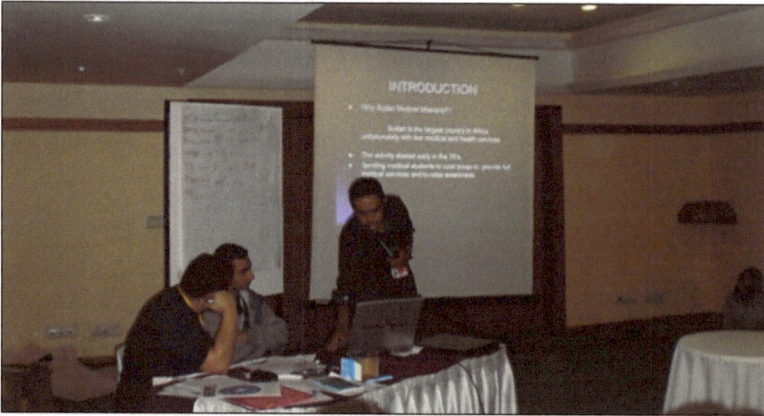

Photo 73: Health Education Secretary (KMSA) and National Public Health Officer (MedSIN-Sudan), Ahmed Hashim (author), presenting SMM project at the 54th GA of IFMSA, in Antalya-Turkey.

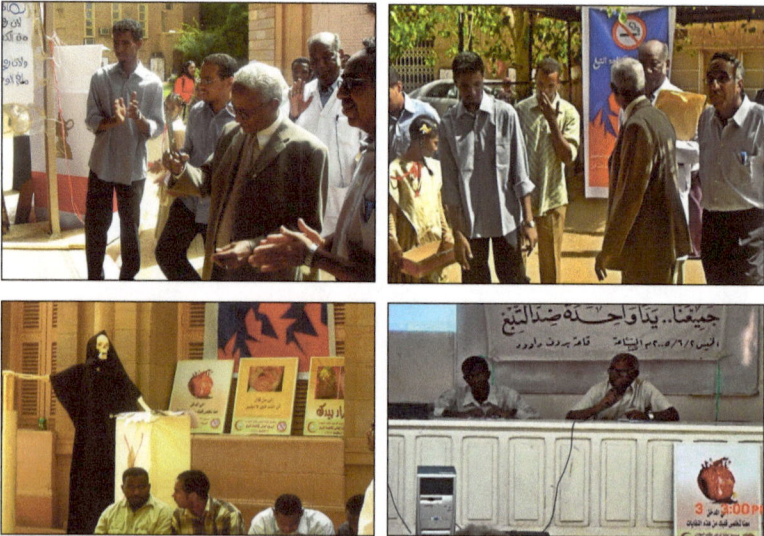

Photo 74: World No Tobacco Day (WNTD), 2005. Standing in the top left image from right to left: Prof. Elbaghir, Prof. Abdelgadir Elkadaro (Faculty Dean, 2003-07), the late Prof. Eldaw Mukhtar (at the back), Ahmed MSK Hashim (Health Education Secretary, the author) and Mohamed Abdelwahab (co-organiser of the day). Bottom-right image: Prof. Elrasheid (Mohamed Elmekki) Ahmed is giving a lecture outlining the deleterious effects of tobacco use.

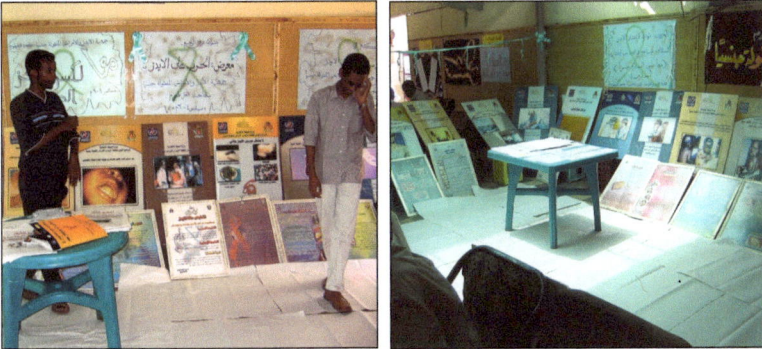

Photo 75: World HIV Day, 2004.

The Secretariat of Media and Culture was chaired by Osman Hassan, who resigned mid-term and was replaced by Hiba Abdalla, who remained in this position until the end of the term. The major achievement of this office was the publication of the Association's news and culture magazine, named *Nabd*, which means "pulse". This focused on the students' talents in literature, poetry and journalism, holding interviews with the faculty staff members, and giving regular updates on student activities. The first editor of *Nabd* was Ahmed Abdelwahid and the front page of the second-edition, edited by Masooma Abdalla is displayed below (**photo 77**). Many cultural sub-societies flourished during this time, covering activities such as poetry and theatre (**photo 76**).

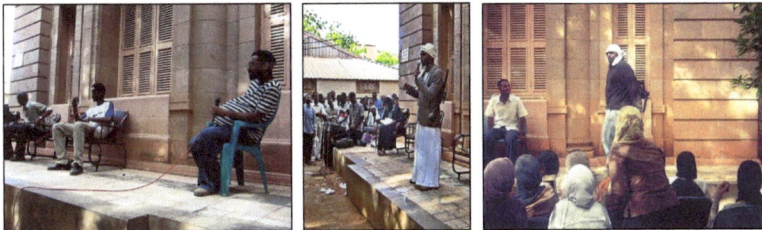

Photo 76: Members of the Theatre Society performing plays at World Peace Day, 2004, and World No Tobacco Day, 2005.

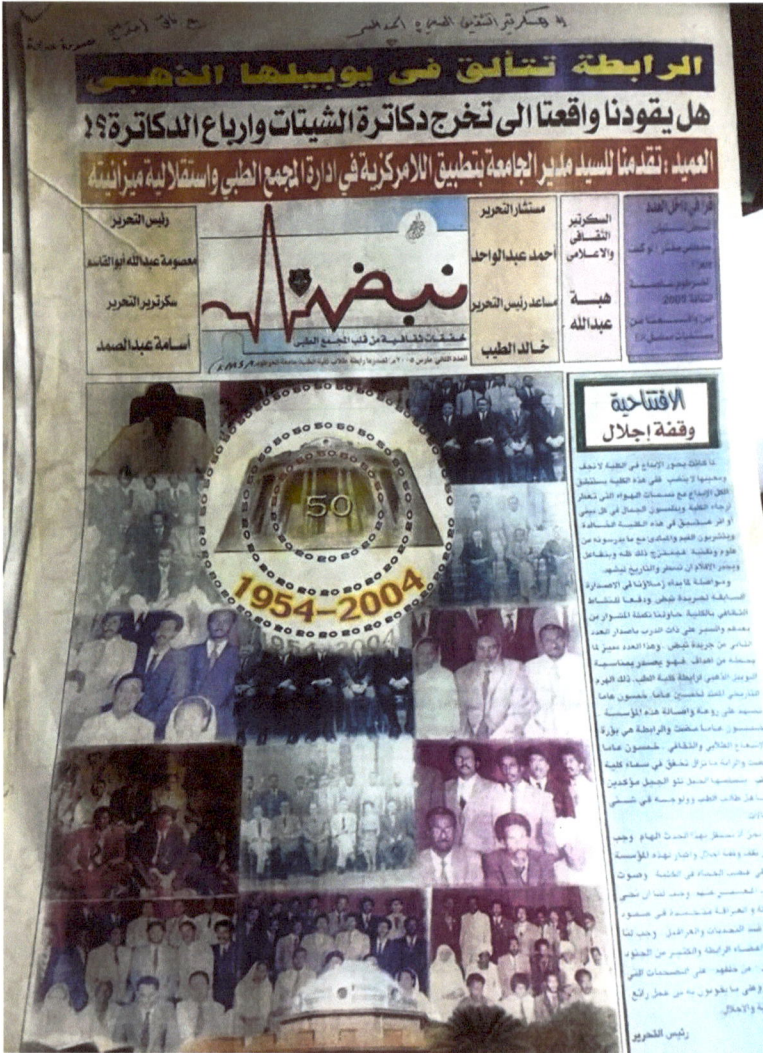

Photo 77: The Golden Jubilee special edition of *Nabd* Magazine. Editor-in-Chief of this issue; Masooma Abdalla. Advisory Editor: Ahmed Abdelwahid.

Mutaz Elsadig and Khalifa Hassan became the Association's Secretary General and Assistant to Secretary General, respectively. Mutaz, who was described by many as the dynamo of the committee, was an active and very articulate member of the executive board and played a pivotal role in writing the different by-laws, representing the Association in many occasions, and co-ordinating the work of the different offices of the executive committee.

The General Secretariat organised many successful activities, including World Peace Day (WPD) in 2004, which was hosted for the first time by the Students' Association. The on-going conflicts in Darfur were intensifying at that time and a celebration of WPD was deemed a priority by the group in view of this. Hence, the event was given the theme *'We are all for Darfur'* and included a war/peace exhibition, plus internal student broadcasting and theatre performances (**photo 78**). Donations were also collected to aid vulnerable people in Darfur refugee camps.

The Association also hosted an open day in the faculty to show solidarity with the victims of the tsunami in Indonesia and South-East Asia. The exhibition of this event is shown below (**photos 79**).

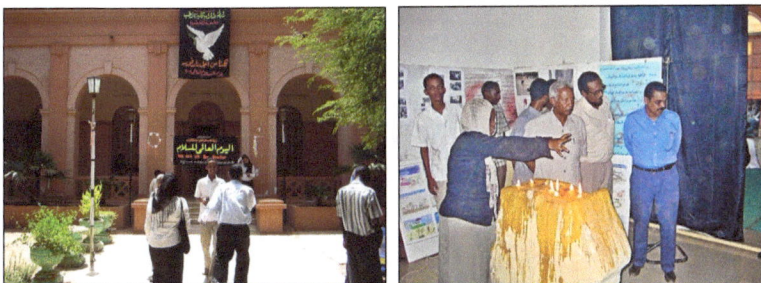

Photo 78: World Peace Day, 2004. On the right, from right to left: Dr. Essam Elkhidir, Prof. Mustafa Idris, and Prof. Abdelgadir Elkadaro (Faculty Dean).

Internationally, the team made remarkable achievements through MedSIN-Sudan. Maha Elamin, the Secretary of External Affairs, worked closely with President Ahmed Eltahir, to expand the scope of MedSIN-Sudan. Ahmed Eltahir also made enormous efforts, leading to the introduction of the new constitution, making contact with different medical students' associations and enhancing

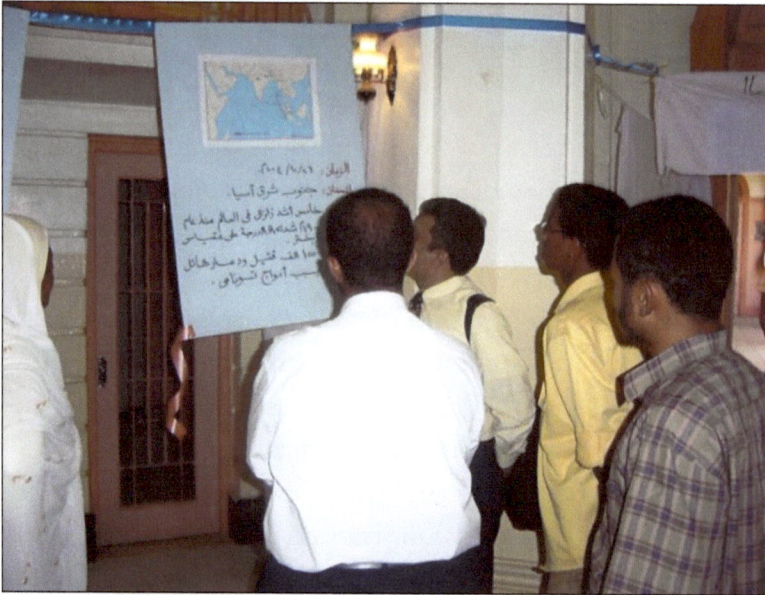

Photo 79: The tsunami aid exhibition, 2004-05.

the membership of MedSIN-Sudan, to transform it into a true umbrella organisation for all the medical students in Sudan.

Following adoption of the new constitution, MedSIN-Sudan had its first official international debut at the 54th IFMSA GA in Antalya-Turkey, with a delegation of over ten students, with a representative in each of the IFMSA standing committees. In addition to medical students from the KMSA, the delegation included representatives from Ahfad and Bakht Elrida Medical Students' Associations (**photo 80**). The participation of this Sudanese delegation in that meeting resulted in new cross-organization collaborations and more opportunities for the Students' Exchange Programme. More importantly, the team presented the proposal of Sudan Village Concept Project (VCP) 3 at the meeting's plenary session (**photo 80**).

The Sudan VCP-3 had in fact, been proposed before the return of the Association in 2003, but could not be initiated in the 2004-05 term, mainly due to funding limitations. However, the team managed to finalise and present a well-designed proposal for the project and the VCP-3 was set to take place in Al-Gezira state, in an area consisting of eleven villages, called *Al-Agalyen*. In the end, this was narrowed to a field of four villages in that area. The project had a total budget of 310,000 euros and received support from the U of K Department of Community Medicine, and the Sudan Development Call Organisation (*Nidaa*).

The objectives of Sudan VCP-3 were to:

- Decrease the incidence of diarrhea in children below five years.
- Decrease the incidence of respiratory tract infections.
- Increase the villager's knowledge about major endemic diseases especially Malaria and Bilharzia.
- Construct a health center (to the WHO health center standard with extended services)
- Establish a drug supply system.
- Achieve 90% coverage of the vaccination for the six killer diseases of childhood.
- Raise the access to public latrines from 84% to 100%.
- Establish a garbage disposal system.
- Raise the community awareness about oral hygiene.
- Improve meat inspection services to ensure a good quality of offered products; follow up prevailing disease in animals and prevent further spreading to consumers.
- Improve and increase agricultural productivity rate of field crops (sorghum, wheat, and groundnut).
- Enlarge the water stations' capacity at each village from 30.8% to 75.00% of the total needs for each resident.
- Increase the mothers' knowledge and usage of Oral Rehydration Solutions from 37.2% to 80%.

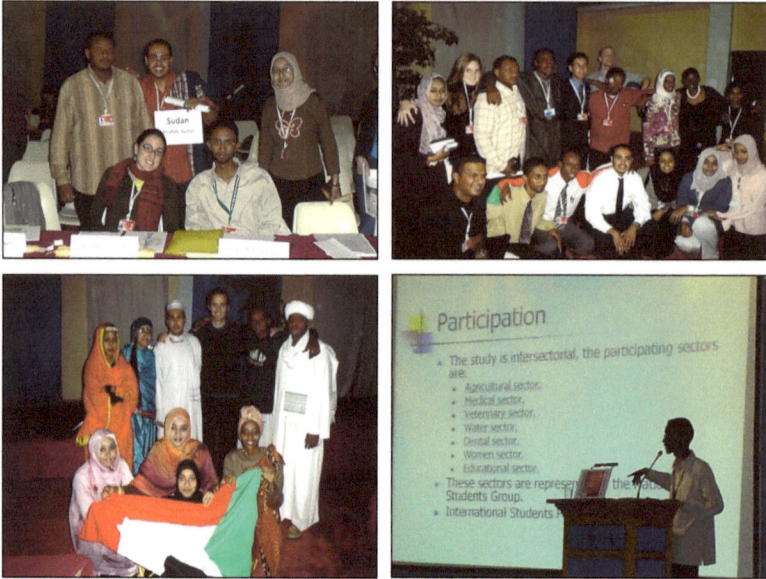

Photo 80: MedSIN-Sudan delegation at the 54th IFMSA GA in Antalya, Turkey, 2005. Bottom right: KMSA President Ahmed Eltahir presents the proposal of Sudan Village Concept Project 3 (VCP-3) at the plenary session of the meeting.

At the following IFMSA GA in Egypt, President Ahmed Eltahir was elected as the IFMSA Regional Coordinator of Africa, 2005-06 and was then nominated at the Serbia IFMSA August Meeting (2006) for the position of IFMSA President for 2006-07. He subsequently become the first Sudanese and Middle Eastern medical student to be elected President of the IFMSA and his election to these two prestigious IFMSA roles (African Coordinator and President) is still considered one of the KMSA's major successes at the international level (**photo 81**).

MedSIN-Sudan held its first GA under the new constitution in 2005, at the Faculty of Medicine, University of Khartoum. Nearly ten medical students' associations participated and many workshops were conducted in the various offices (**photo 82**). The group invited Emily Spry, the ex-President of the IFMSA (2003-04), who kindly accepted and made a historic visit to Sudan in 2005. Together with Audun Melaas, a professional trainer from Norway, she organised and delivered the first student Train New Trainers (TNT) workshop (**photo 83**).

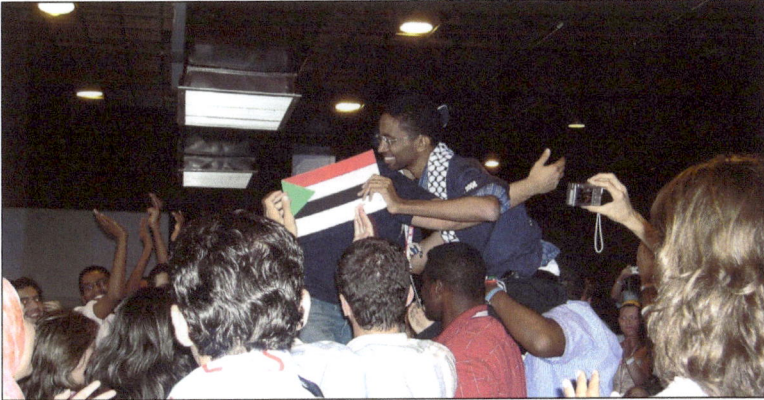

Photo 81: Ahmed Eltahir, lifted on the shoulders by African and Middle-eastern students following his historical election as IFMSA president at the GA in Serbia, 2006.

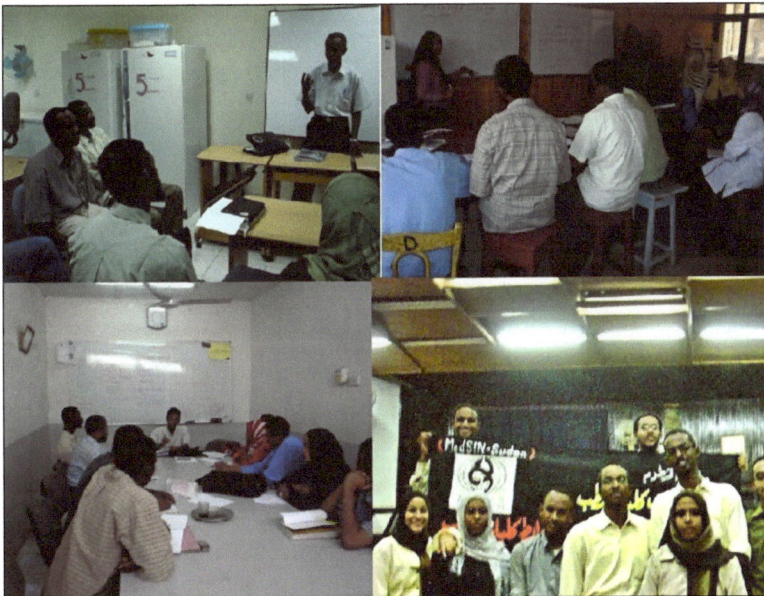

Photo 82: Some of the activities at MedSIN-Sudan GA, 2005.

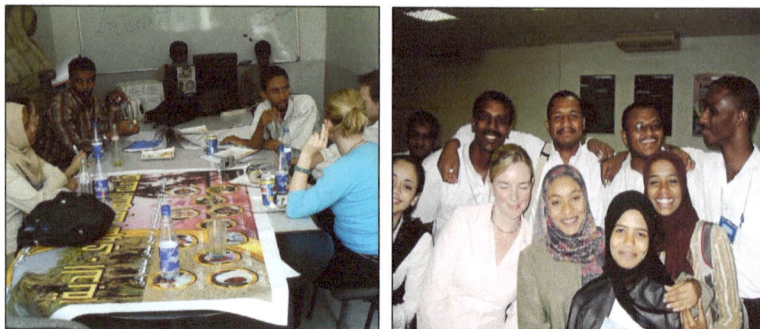

Photo 83: Train New Trainers (TNT) Workshop and Emily Spry's visit to Khartoum. Right-hand image, front row second from the left: Emily Spry, ex-President of the IFMSA, 2003-2004.

Prior to introducing the new MedSIN-Sudan constitution, the group also attended the FAMSA regional scientific meeting in Ibadan, Nigeria, which was themed *War, AIDS and the African Child*. The delegation included President Ahmed Eltahir, Mutaz Elsadig, Ahmed MSK Hashim (The author), and Mohamed Abdelghani (**photo 84**). Sadly, the meeting was not well attended, with students from only three countries present (Nigeria, Sudan, and Ghana), despite the organisers claiming that thirteen countries had sent confirmation of attendance. Moreover, it was discovered that FAMSA had not held regular GAs over the preceding years, due to disagreements between the members, which resulted in a boycott of FAMSA by many African countries; the last GA was held in Nigeria in 2001. The KMSA delegation was surprised to learn that the Vice-President of FAMSA at that time was Majok Malek, a Sudanese medical student from Bahr-Elghazal University who was elected in 2001. According to the FAMSA constitution, as the Vice-President, Majok was supposed to host the next FAMSA GA in Sudan but for unknown reasons the GA was not held. After this regional FAMSA meeting in Ibadan, the KMSA delegation realized these conflicts were weakening the organisation and consequently, the group diverted their attention to the African division of the IFMSA.

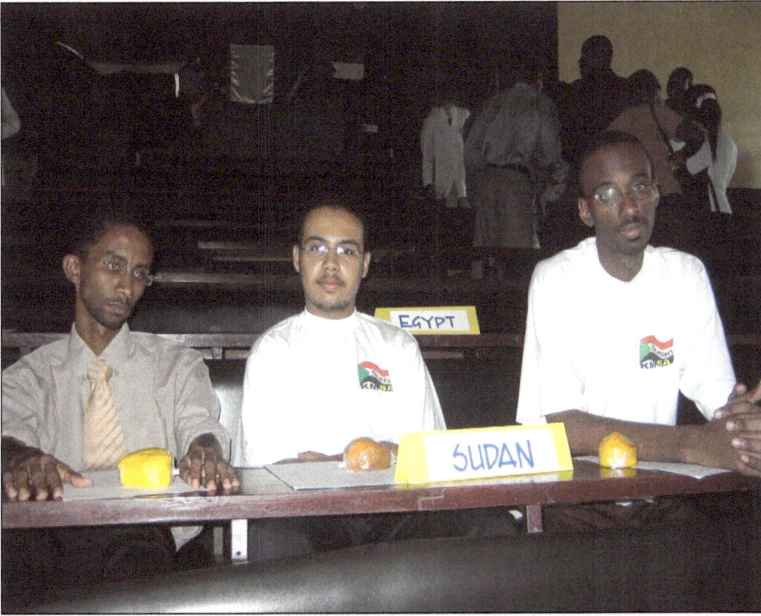

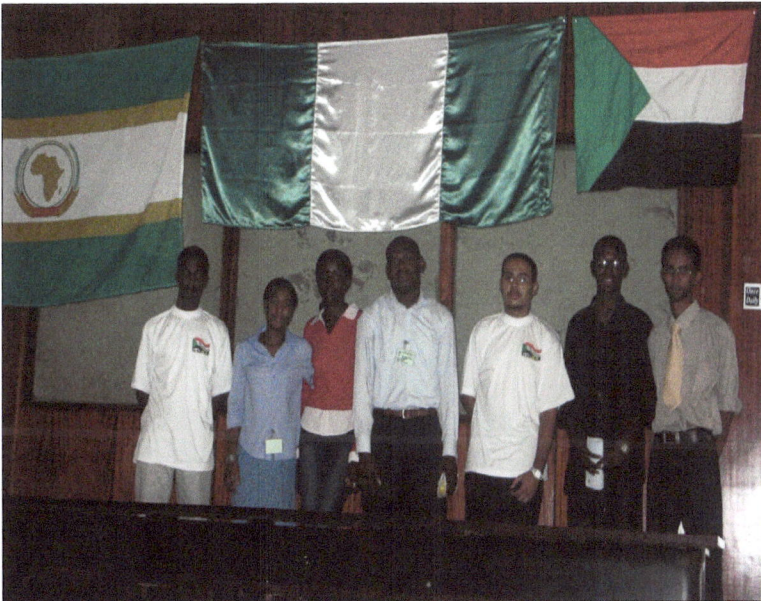

Photo 84: The delegation of the KMSA at the regional meeting of the FAMSA in Ibadan, Nigeria, 2004. Upper image, seated left to right: Ahmed Eltahir, Ahmed MSK Hashim (author), and Mutaz Elsadig.

The Golden Jubilee
of the Association
(1954 – 2004)

The key event organised by the General Secretariat for 2004-05 was the Golden Jubilee Celebration, marking the 50th anniversary of the Association. Celebrations took place in March 2005. Prior to that day, the executive board launched a documentation campaign to gather information about the history of the KMSA and its activities and the author was assigned to be head of the Documentation and Archiving Committee. Many interviews were held with previous Association presidents and detailed written accounts of the Association's activities were submitted by previous members via email. Photos of the Association's activities were also collected, identified, and labelled.

The Golden Jubilee event was co-organised by Mutaz Elsadig and the author, Ahmed MSK Hashim. Together, they produced the programme for the day, invited the guests, and designed the History of KMSA exhibition/Museum (**photo 85**). In addition, fourth-year medical students played a pivotal role in the success of the event namely, Haytham Essam, Sami Elamin (member of the council and President of the following term 2005-06), Elmahi, Hussam Hamad, Wael Gorafi, Musaab Wahbani, Abdalla Enayat and Nihal Omer. The event included an exhibition of the history of the KMSA and a session on KMSA's history, led by past presidents, plus an evening programme. All attending ex-presidents were honoured and given dedication plaques. Among the presidents who attended the event were: Mirghani Ahmed Abdelaziz, Ahmed Elsafi, Tarig Ismail, Haydar Giha, Abdelrahman Ali, Abdelrahman Musa, Osman Mohamed Ahmed Taha, and Haddad Karoum.

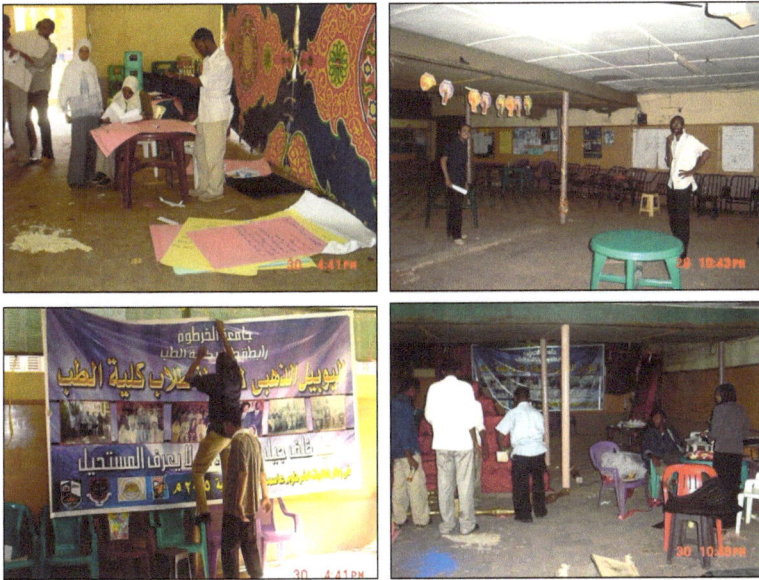

Photo 85: Members of the KMSA's Golden Jubilee organising committee preparing for the celebrations and the history museum, 2005.

The speakers session was chaired by Mutaz Elsadig with the author acting as facilitator. Ahmed Eltahir spoke about the return of the Association and the role of medical students in the development of health services while ex-presidents Haydar Giha, Mirghani A. Abdelaziz, Ahmed Elsafi and Tarig Ismail described their experiences during their respective terms in office (**photo 87**).

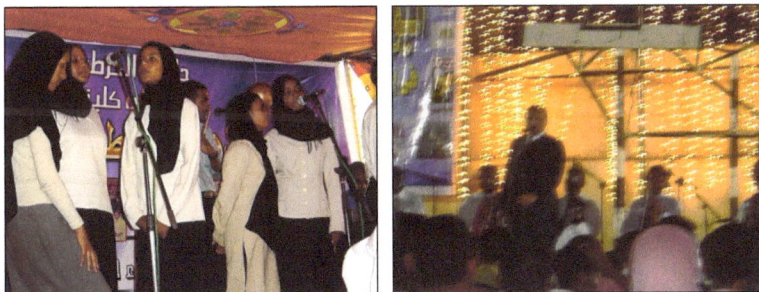

Photo 86: On the left: The Students' Choir performing at the Golden Jubilee event. On the right: Musician Hafiz Abdelrahman performing at the evening programme and dinner in Awad Omer Elsammani Stadium, 2005.

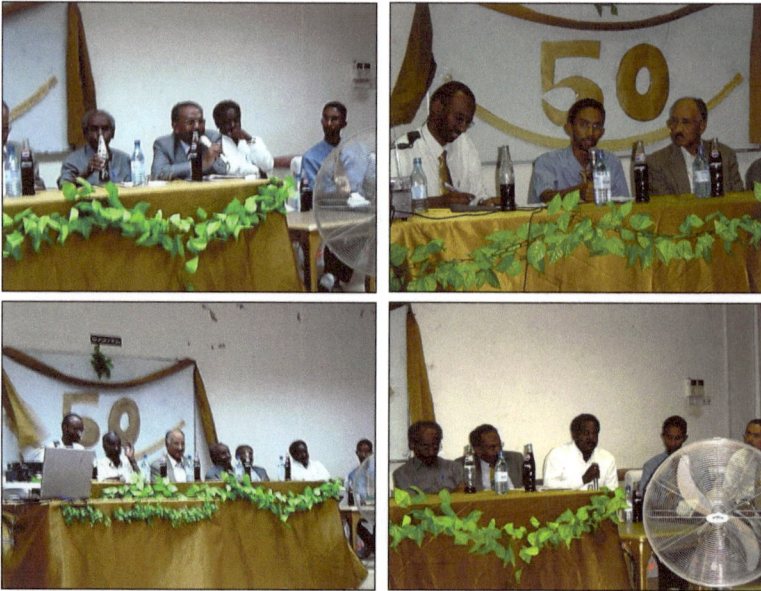

Photo 87: The History of the KMSA session, Prof. Daoud Lecture Theatre, 2005. Bottom-left photo, from left to right: Mutaz Elsadig (Secretary General, 2004-05), Prof. Abdelrahman Musa (President, 1960-61), Dr Mirghani A. Abdelaziz (President, 1966-67), Prof. Ahmed Elsafi (President, 1970-71), Mr. Tarig Ismail (President, 1976-77), Prof. Haydar Giha (President, 1987-88), Ahmed Eltahir (President, 2004-05).

The performance by the Students' Choir was the highlight of the evening programme as well as a flute solo by musician Hafiz Abdulrahman (**photo 86**). The Faculty Dean, Abdelgadir Elkadaro, gave a speech at the end of the evening dinner which addressed the role of the faculty in promoting students' welfare.

The photos overleaf (**88, 89, 90**) show part of the Golden Jubilee exhibition, the KMSA museum, and the ceremony honouring the KMSA's previous presidents.

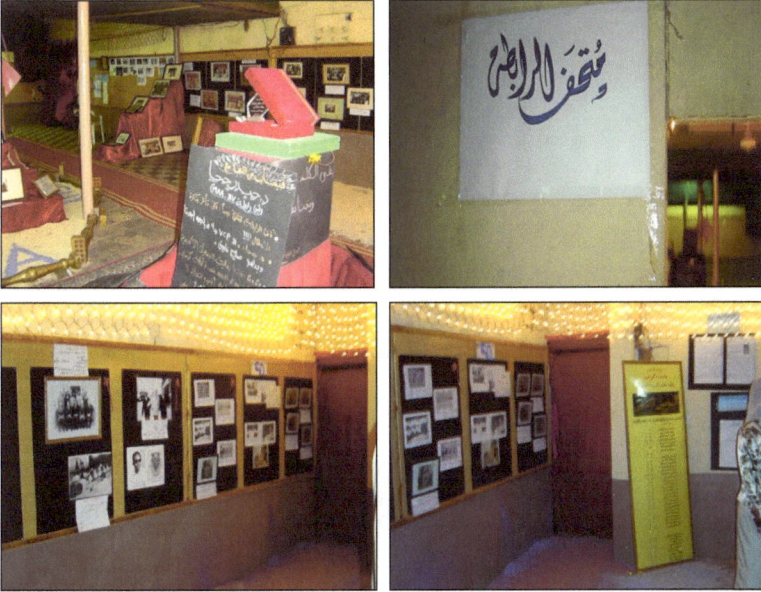

مُتحَفّ الراهي

Photo 88: KMSA History Museum – Golden Jubilee celebrations, 2005.

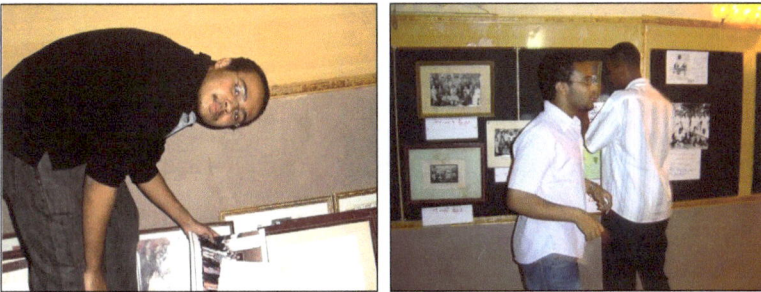

Photo 89: Preparations of the KMSA history museum, 2005. Left-hand image: Ahmed Hashim (author), head of documentation and archiving committee. Right-hand image: students Zuhair Tarig (left) and Gassan Abdelsalam (right).

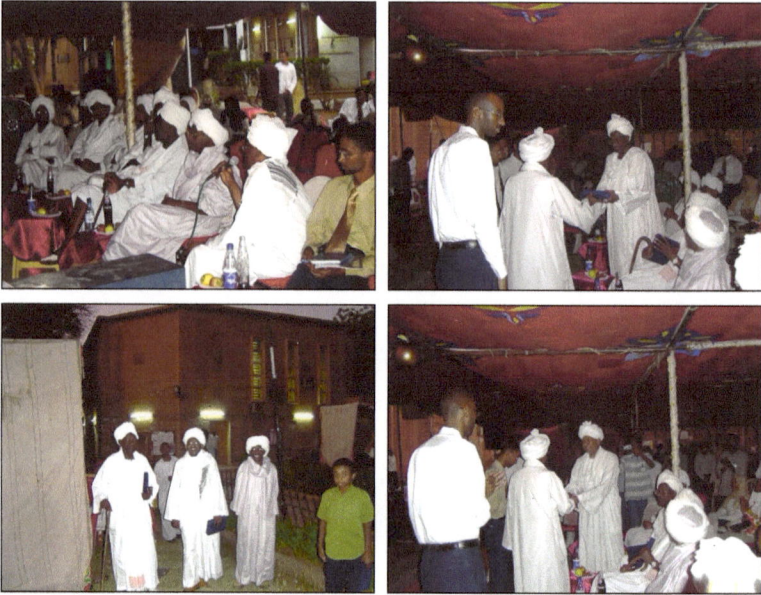

Photo 90: Honouring the previous presidents of the Association at the Golden Jubilee event, 2005.

References

Al Hakeem Journal. No.16. 1964

Al Hakeem Journal. No.17. 1964

Al Hakeem Journal. No.19. 1965

Al Hakeem Journal. No 21. 1966.

Al Hakeem Journal. Vol.7 no.1. 1968

Al Hakeem Journal. No.23. 1968

Al Hakeem Journal. Vol.7. 1969.

Al Hakeem Journal. Vol. 8 no.1. 1970.

Al Hakeem Journal. Vol. 8 no.2. 1971

Al Hakeem Journal. Vol.9, no2. 1974

Al Hakeem Journal. Vol. 11, no. 2. 1977

Al Hakeem Journal. Vol. 12 no.2. 1978

Daoud Mustafa Khalid, his life and work (2009) by Ahmed Elsafi

Diaries And Opinions Of A Doctor (translated title) by Prof. Salih
Yassin. مذكرات طبيب وآراء

El Hakeim Journal. Vol. 1 no.1. 1957

El Hakeim Journal. Vol. 1 no.2. 1957

El Hakeim Journal. Vol. 1 no.3. 1958

El Hakeim Journal. Vol. 1 no.4. 1958

El Hakeim Journal. Vol. 1 no.5. 1958

El Hakeim Journal. Vol. 1 no.6. 1959

El Hakeim Journal. Vol. 1 no.9. 1960

Faculty of Medicine – University of Khartoum 1924 -1999 – Translated title- ("The Diamond Jubilee Book") by Ezzan Saeed. ١٩٩٩ -١٩٢٤ جامعة الخرطوم ـ كلية الطب

Faculty of Medicine – University of Khartoum website. http://meduofk.net/ (Accessed 28/05/2017)

Federation of African Medical Students' Association (FAMSA) thru the years (1968 -2015) booklet.

Federation of African Medical Students' Association (FAMSA) website. http://famsanet.org/ (Accessed 28/05/2017).

Genital Mutilation of Girls in Sudan Community- and hospital-based studies on female genital cutting and its sequelae by Lars Almroth. Karolinska University Press, 2005.

International Federation of Medical Students' Associations (IFMSA) Website. https://ifmsa.org/ (Accessed 28/05/2017)

International Federation of Medical Students' Associations (IFMSA) 60th anniversary (1951 – 2011) booklet.

International Federation of Medical Students' Associations (IFMSA) annual reports (1993-2000).

KMSA Archives (with permission from steering committee 2016-2017).

Salih MAM. Remembering for tomorrow: Professor Mansour Ali Haseeb. *Sudanese Journal of Paediatrics.* 2013;13(2):76-83.

Tigani al-Mahi: The Father of African Psychiatry. Introduction, In: Ahmad Al-Safi; Taha Baasher, Editors. Tigani El Mahi: Selected Essays. Ist. Ed. Khartoum: Khartoum University Press; 1984

Appendix 1:

Association Presidents List

Association President	Term	رئيس الرابطة
Mohamed Ahmed Gabani	54-55	محمد أحمد قباني
Haddad Omer Karoum	55-56	حداد عمر كروم
Hassan Mohamed Ibrahim	56-57	حسن محمد إبراهيم
Mohamed Abdelaziz Abusamra	57-58	محمد عبدالعزيز أبو سمرة
Kamal Zaki Mustafa	58-59	كمال زكي مصطفى
Musa Abdalla Hamid	59-60	موسى عبدالله حامد
Abdelrahman Musa	60-61	عبدالرحمن محمد موسى
Salah Taha Salih	61-62	صلاح طه صالح
Hassan Osman Omer	62-63	حسن عثمان عمر
Mohamed Zain	63-64	محمد زين محمد (أحمد)
Osman Mohamed Ahmed Taha	64-65	عثمان محمد أحمد طه
Ali Elhaj Mohamed	65-66	علي الحاج محمد

English	Year	Arabic
Mirghani Ahmed Abdelaziz	66-67	ميرغني أحمد عبد العزيز
Abdelsalam Gerais	67-68	عبد السلام جريس
Hassan Fadlalla	68-69	حسن فضل الله
Ahmed Ibrahim Mukhtar	69-70	أحمد ابراهيم مختار
Ahmed Elsafi	70-71	أحمد الصافي
Omer Ibrahim Aboud	71-72	عمر ابراهيم عبود
Mohamed Elmahdi Balla	72-73	محمد المهدي بلة
Abdelrahman Ali	73-74	عبد الرحمن علي
Abdalmagid Mohamed Musaad	74-75	عبد الماجد محمد مساعد
Bakri Osman Saeed (Beginning of term)	75-76	بكري عثمان سعيد
Balla Mohamed Elbashir	75-76	بلة محمد البشير
Tarig Ismail Humaida	76-77	طارق إسماعيل حميدة
Abdelhaleem Elhidai	77-78	عبد الحليم الهداي
Ahmed Farah Shadoul	78-79	أحمد فرح شادول
Aasim Sidahmed Yousif	79-80	عاصم سيد أحمد يوسف
Awad Osman (Abu Sheiba)	80-81	عوض عثمان (أبو شيبة)
Abdelrahman Almubarak	81-82	عبد الرحمن المبارك أك عثمان
Abdelhadi Abdelgabbar Abdelhadi	82-83	عبدالهادي عبدالجبار عبدالهادي

Ahmed Abdelrahim Elbashir	83-84	أحمد عبد الرحيم البشير
Abdelbagi Ahmed Abdelbagi	84-85	عبدالباقي أحمد عبدالباقي
Osama Awad Mohamed Jaafar	85-86	اسامة عوض محمد جعفر
Nadir Khogali	86-87	نادر خوجلي
Haydar Ahmed Giha	87-88	حيدر أحمد جحا
Hamdeen Hammad Hamdeen	88-89	حامدين حماد حامدين
Baheldin Abbas Badawi	89-90	بهاء الدين عباس بدوي
Essam Eldin Elamin	90-91	عصام الدين الأمين
Elsadig Askar	91-92	الصادق عسكر

The Association officially suspended

Elmonzir Bajouri	03-04	المنذر باجوري
Ahmed Eltahir Osman	04-05	أحمد الطاهر عثمان

121

Appendix 2:

Important Milestones in the History of KMSA

Year	Highlight
1954	The KMSA established as Students' Medical Society (SMS)
1957	First print edition of *Al Hakeem* (*El Hakeim*) published
1960-61	The society creates its own bank account
1966	The Society requests to joins the IFMSA
1967	The Society attains full IFMSA membership and begins to participate in the professional exchange programme
1967	The Society becomes the Medical Students' Association (MSA)
1967	IFMSA president Mr Ian Fraser visits Khartoum and meets members of the MSA

1968	The first bibliographical index of *Al Hakeem* compiled
1974 – 75	Gaafer Mohamed Fageir becomes FAMSA's SCOH director
1978-79	Ahmed F. Shadoul becomes FAMSA's President
1981	First official representation of medical students from the MSA in the IFMSA board (Abdelrahman Almubarak becomes SCOPA director)
1981-84	Sudan Medical Students Association (SMSA) allows AlGezira, Juba medical students to join.
1982	Mohyeldin Mohamed Ali becomes IFMSA's SCOPH director
1988	The Association contributed significantly in the aid operations during the 1988 floods
1990-91	The Association pharmacy opened
1991	Prof. Omer Beleil Audio-Visual centre established
1991	The Association was officially suspended
1993	Khalid Mohamed Eltahir becomes IFMSA's SCOR director
1994	Mohamed Abdulgabbar Ahmed becomes SCORP director

1994	Sudan VCP -1 began
1998	Sudan VCP-2 began
1999-2000	Medical students participate in the Faculty's Diamond Jubilee
2003	MedSIN Sudan created (replacing SMSA)
2003	The return of the Association as KMSA
2006-07	Ahmed Eltahir becomes IFMSA president

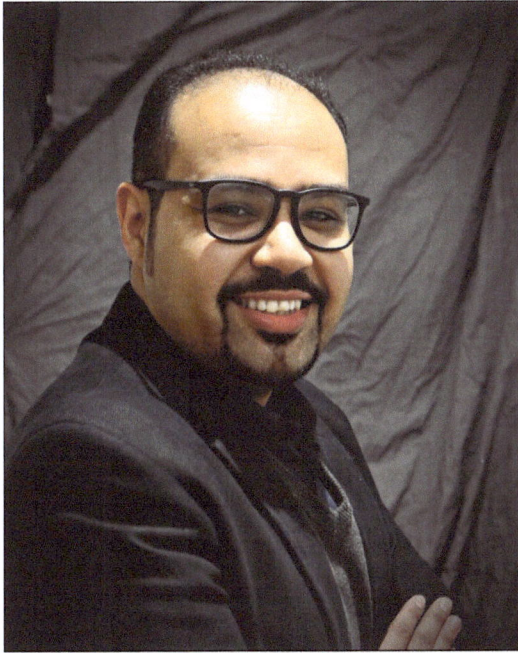

Dr Ahmed MSK Hashim (MBBS, MRCP (UK), MSc, FHEA) is currently working as a gastroenterology & hepatology trainee in the UK. He obtained MBBS from the Faculty of Medicine-University of Khartoum in 2008, having served as a member of the executive committee of the Khartoum Medical Students' Association (KMSA) between 2004 & 2005, when he was also the chair of the Documentation Committee of the Association. Dr Hashim has always been interested in the history of the extracurricular activities of the medical students of University of Khartoum since that time.

Roles Held by the Author in Medical School:

- Head of the second-year Innovation Day 2003

- Member of the representative committee for batch 79, 2003-04

- Member of the Khartoum Medical Students' Association (KMSA) council 2004-05

- Member of the executive committee of KMSA 2004-05

- Health Education Secretary KMSA 2004-05

- National Public Officer for MedSIN-Sudan 2004-05

- ***Head of the Documentation & Archiving Committee 2004-05***

- Coordinator of the World Peace Day celebrations 2004

- Coordinator of KMSA's Golden Jubilee Celebrations 2005

- Organizer of the World No Tobacco day, 2005.

www.ingramcontent.com/pod-product-compliance
Lightning Source LLC
Chambersburg PA
CBHW041314210326
41599CB00008B/265